Reiner Bartl · Bertha Frisch

OSTEOPOROSIS
Diagnosis, Prevention, Therapy

**A Practical Guide for all Physicians –
from Pediatrics to Geriatrics**

With 75 Figures and 25 Tables

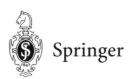

Springer

ISBN 3-540-40499-6 Springer-Verlag Berlin Heidelberg New York

Cataloging-in-Publication Data applied for
Bibliographic information published by Die Deutsche Bibliothek. Die Deutsche
Bibliothek lists this publication in the Deutsche Nationalbibliografie; detailed bib-
liographic data is available in the Internet at <http://dnb.ddb.de>.

Springer-Verlag is a part of Springer Science + Business Media
springeronline.com

© Springer-Verlag Berlin Heidelberg 2004
Printed in Germany

Illustrations: R. Henkel, Heidelberg
Cover design: E. Kirchner, Heidelberg
Product management and layout: B. Wieland, Heidelberg
Typesetting: AM-production, Wiesloch
Printing and bookbinding: Mercedes-Druck, Berlin

24/3150 – 5 4 3 2 1 0
Printed on acid-free paper

Authors

Reiner Bartl
Professor of Internal Medicine,
Osteology, Hematology and Oncology
Department of Internal Medicine III
Bavarian Center of Osteoporosis
University of Munich
Germany

Bertha Frisch
Professor of Hematology
Departments of Pathology and Hematology
Sourasky Medical Center
University of Tel Aviv
Israel

Christoph Bartl, MD
Department of Trauma-,
Hand- and Reconstructive Surgery
University of Ulm
Germany

Preface

With the dawn of the 21st century has come the realisation that bone and joint diseases are the major cause of pain and physical disability worldwide. It is undoubtedly this insight that prompted the WHO to declare the first 10 years of the new century as "The Bone and Joint Decade 2000–2010". The number of people suffering from these diseases – already many millions in every so-called developed as well as underdeveloped country in the world – is expected to double within the next 20 years. In many countries the increase will be even greater due to the longer survival and consequently larger numbers of older people in the population. It is inevitable that the already astronomical costs of health care will rise proportionally.

On the positive side there is also no doubt that the enormous amount of work and research on disorders of bone over the past 10–20 years or so has contributed greatly to our understanding of their causes, treatment and prevention. Most importantly, perhaps, the skeleton is now regarded in a new light: as a dynamic organ undergoing constant renewal throughout life from start to finish, from the cradle to the grave. What is more, it is now abundantly clear that the skeleton participates in almost every condition that may effect the body!

This applies especially to osteoporosis, which, as emphasised by the title of this book, is now under control! How did this come about?

▶ Because of the elucidation of the factors involved in osseous remodelling.
▶ Because of the development of simple, fast, reliable and non-invasive methods for measurement of bone density.
▶ Because of the identification of risk factors to which everybody is exposed, so that appropriate measures can be taken to prevent development of osteoporosis and/or its progression when fractures have already occurred.

▶ And because effective medication for prevention and therapy is now readily available worldwide.

The efficacy of the classes of compounds known as the bisphosphonates as well as the "selective oestrogen receptor modulators" (SERMs) and parathyroid hormones has now been unequivocally established by numerous large multicentre trials involving literally millions of patients. In addition, simple methods such as a healthy life-style, adequate nutrition, sufficient physical activity, vitamin D and calcium supplements as required can be recommended and adopted on a large scale. Introduction and acceptance of these methods requires public awareness and support and the realisation that every individual is the guardian and caretaker of his/her own bones and responsible for their structural integrity. Still lacking, however, is widespread recognition of these facts both among the public at large but more importantly among members of the medical profession. To day, at the start of the new millennium, when information and knowledge are freely available, such a state of affairs cannot be tolerated. Well-established diagnostic techniques and effective therapies – both antiresorptive and osteoanabolic – are now available for prevention, diagnosis and treatment of osteoporosis. It should be emphasized that the treatments recommended in this text are all founded on "Evidence based Medicine" (unless otherwise stated) for which the appropriate references are given at the end of the text.

The aim of this book is to demonstrate that bone is everybody's business and especially every doctor's, and to provide guidelines for the diagnosis, therapy and prevention of osteoporosis – from paediatrics to geriatrics. This book will raise awareness and inform physicians across disciplines about this preventable and now also treatable disease.

Our particular goal has been to make this text as "user-friendly" as possible so that any doctor seeking information on a particular topic in osteoporosis has uncomplicated and time-saving access to it.

We wish all our readers success in their endeavours to help patients and to reduce suffering on this strife-ridden, beautiful planet of ours. God bless you all!

REINER BARTL   BERTHA FRISCH
Munich   Tel Aviv

Contents

1 Osteoporosis: An Epidemic of Overwhelming Proportions! 1

Osteoporosis: A Silent Thief 1
Osteoporosis: The Global Scope of the Problem 2

2 Bone: A Fascinating Organ 5

Bone: An Architectural Masterpiece 5
Bone: A Permanent Building and Rebuilding Site 9
Control of Bone Remodelling:
   A Network of Complex Mechanisms. 16
Leptin: Role of the Central Nervous System
   in Regulation of Bone 20
Peak Bone Mass: An Investment for a Healthier Life. 22

3 Definition of Osteoporosis 24

Osteoporosis: How to Define it 24
Osteoporosis: Which Bones Are Vulnerable 26
Osteoporosis: Also a Question of Quality. 27
How to Define "Fracture"? Not So Simple! 29

4 Subgroups of Osteoporosis: From Different Points of View 33

According to Spread 33
According to Sex and Age 35
According to Extent 37
According to Histology. 38

5 Recognition of Risk Factors 40

Risk Factors Which Cannot (Yet) Be Influenced 40
Risk Factors Which Can Be Influenced 43

6 Clinical Investigations in Osteoporosis 49

Symptoms 49
Osteoporosis and Teeth, Skin, and Hair 52
Role of Conventional X-Rays 53
Other Useful Imaging Techniques 55

7 Bone Mineral Density (BMD): The Crucial Diagnostic Parameter . . 58

Why Measure Bone Mineral Density? 58
Which Instruments to Use? 60
Which Bones to Measure? 66
Indications for BMD 68
Bone Densitometry in Children: Now Readily Available 71
BMD Measurement: Not a Scary Procedure,
    Nothing to Be Afraid of! 71

8 Laboratory Investigations in Osteoporosis: Are They Needed? . . . 73

Which Tests Are Necessary? 73
Significance of Markers of Bone Turnover 75
When Is a Bone Biopsy Indicated? 79

9 Preventive Care for Lifelong Healthy Bones 80

Step 1: A Calcium-Rich Diet 80
Step 2: An Adequate Supply of Vitamins 84
Step 3: Protect the Spine in Everyday Living 85
Step 4: Regular Physical Activity 87

Step 5: No Smoking   89
Step 6: Reduce Nutritional "Bone Robbers"   90
Step 7: An Ideal Body Weight   93
Step 8: Drugs that Cause Osteoporosis   93
Step 9: Diseases that Damage Bones   95

10 How to Treat Osteoporosis   97

Evidence-Based Medicine for Therapy of Osteoporosis   97
Comprehensive Approach to Therapy of Osteoporosis 103

11 First and Foremost: Management of Pain 105

Treat the Patient, Not Only the Disease 105
Acute Phase 105
Chronic Phase: Short Term 106
Chronic Phase: Long Term 107
Electric Potentials in Bone 107

12 Calcium and Vitamin D: The Skeleton's Best Friends 109

Calcium: A Lifelong Companion, From Infancy Onwards 109
Vitamin D: Don't Rely on Sunshine, Take Supplements 112

13 Hormones for Replacement: A Matter of Re-Evaluation 117

Hormone Replacement Therapy (HRT) for Women:
    Now Recommended Only for Symptoms
    and for Short Periods Only 117
Natural Oestrogens: How Effective Are They? 123
Dehydroepiandrosterone (DHEA):
    Is It Useful for Prevention of Bone Loss? 126
Testosterone: Good for Bones and Well-being in Men 126
Anabolic Steroids: Strong Muscles for Healthy Bones 127

14 Bisphosphonates: The Success Story in Osteoporosis 128

A Brief Survey of Bisphosphonates 129
Pharmacokinetics 134
Toxicity and Contraindications 135
Bisphosphonates Currently Used in Osteoporosis 137
Long-term Follow-up Studies 141
Monitoring the Effects of Bisphosphonates 142
Nonresponders to Bisphosphonates: Do They Exist? 143

15 Raloxifene: A Potent Selective Oestrogen
Receptor Modulator (SERM) 145

A Brief Survey of SERMs: New Selective Antiresorptive Agents . . 145
Raloxifene: Utilisation of Physiological Effects on Bone 145

16 Parathormone: A Promising Osteoanabolic Agent 148

Osteoanabolic Action: Paradoxical Effects
    Depend on Type of Administration 148

17 Additional Medications 151

Calcitonin and Fluoride: No Longer First Line Therapy 151
Other Medications in Use or Under Investigation 152

18 Osteoporotic Fractures Can Be Treated Successfully
But Should Now Be Avoided 155
In Collaboration with Dr. C. Bartl

Fractures: No Reason to Despair 155
Management of Osteoporotic Fractures 160
Fracture Sites and Their Clinical Significance 161
Aseptic Loosening of Prosthesis 169

19 Osteoporosis: Men Are Also Victims, But With a Time Lag 174

Clinical Evaluation in Men 174
Special Features in Men 177
Prevention and Treatment in Men 178

20 Osteoporosis: Even More Harmful in Children 180

First Clarification: Hereditary or Acquired? 180
Idiopathic Juvenile Osteoporosis (IJO) and Other Conditions . . 185
Osteogenesis Imperfecta (OI) Must Not Be Overlooked 187

21 Osteoporosis: A Danger Lurking in All Medical Disciplines 190

Exclusion of Secondary Osteoporoses:
   A Basic Necessity Before Therapy 190
Cardiology 190
Endocrinology 192
Gastroenterology 192
Genetics 193
Haematology 193
Infectious Disorders (AIDS) 195
Nephrology 195
Neurology 197
Oncology 198
Pulmonology 198
Rheumatology 198

22 Osteoporosis: Many Drugs Are Bone Robbers 199

Corticosteroid-Induced Osteoporosis 199
Transplantation Osteoporosis 204
Tumour Therapy-Induced Osteoporosis 206
Drug-Induced Osteoporomalacia 211

23 Osteoporosis: Unusual Local Manifestations 214

Transient Osteoporosis:
   A Reaction to Local Marrow Inflammation 214
Complex Regional Pain Syndrome (CRPS):
   Reaction to Local Neurostimulation 215
Gorham-Stout Syndrome: The Ultimate Osteoporosis 217

Bibliography 219

Introduction 219
Books on Osteoporosis 219
Selected Articles in Journals 221
Selected Articles Recently Published 229

Subject Index 231

Osteoporosis: An Epidemic of Overwhelming Proportions!

Osteoporosis: A Silent Thief

A young healthy adult can hardly imagine that he/she will ever suffer from osteoporosis. Moreover, when an older individual sustains a fracture or notices a gradual decrease in height, the first reaction is: "This cannot be true, this can't be happening to me. Why should I have osteoporosis? I have never had a single problem with my bones in all my life!" And that is just the problem!

Osteoporosis slowly but surely nibbles away at the bones, possibly unrecognised for years, until finally it is revealed by the occurrence of a fracture almost without cause! And so the vicious circle begins for the patient: fractures – chronic pain – deformities – anger – anxiety – frustration – depression – loss of self-esteem – immobility – and finally social isolation. And the patients are confronted by many psychological, social, and financial problems which at times seem overwhelming. One of the most successful sources of help is the local osteoporosis support group, where patients can learn from others how best to cope with their new challenges. Unfortunately, people are not being educated about the risks of this disease, and people at risk are not receiving preventive information or treatment. Estimates suggest that less than 30 % of women with osteoporosis are diagnosed correctly, and less than 15 % of those diagnosed receive effective treatment. The situation is even worse for men!

Many doctors regard osteoporosis as a "normal" relatively unimportant aspect of the ageing process which can hardly be influenced by outside intervention. Not true – we no longer have to accept osteoporosis as a "normal component" of ageing, which impinges on or even ruins the active life of more than half of all women over 50 years and nearly as many men over 70. The purpose of this book is to unmask this thief and provide the information required for early prevention, correct diagnosis and successful treatment of osteoporosis.

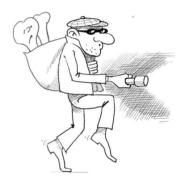

Achieving and maintaining bone health is a lifelong responsibility for all of us.

Osteoporosis is a "silent" risk factor for fracture, just as hypertension is for stroke.

Osteoporosis: The Global Scope of the Problem

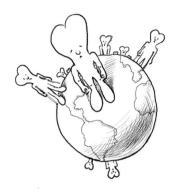

Still global today – but can be eradicated tomorrow.

Today experts have finally come to the realisation that osteoporosis can effect everybody, independent of sex and age. Twenty-five per cent of cases of osteoporosis and fractures now occur in men. Exceptional progress has been made in fundamental research on osteoporosis, its diagnosis, and therapy. *Osteoporosis is now identified as one of the most important diseases affecting the human race*, along with hypertension and diabetes mellitus. For example, an estimated 30 million people suffer from it in the USA, and equally high percentages of the population in European and other countries. While every eighth woman suffers from breast cancer, every third woman sustains a fracture due to osteoporosis. Seventy per cent of the 1.3 million fractures that occur annually in the USA in patients aged 45 years or older are attributable to osteoporosis. From the age of 50 years a woman has the following risk for a fracture:

▶ Vertebral 32 %
▶ Lower arm 16 %
▶ Hip 15 %

Osteoporotic fractures affect more women than heart attacks, strokes and all female cancers combined. Primarily through complications stemming from hip fractures, osteoporosis kills an estimated 50,000 Americans annually, most of them women. Fifty percent of patients with osteoporosis and hip fractures lose their independence. Don't become a victim, prevent osteoporosis and enjoy life instead!

Today in the new millennium it is completely unacceptable that half of all postmenopausal women should suffer fractures when these can be avoided by adequate preventive measures. Furthermore, a hip fracture poses an increased risk of mortality related to coexisting diseases such as stroke, heart failure, or chronic lung diseases, as well as to complications secondary to surgical treatment of the fracture. Nearly 50 % of individuals with hip fractures never fully recover the mobility and independence they had previously, and an additional 25 % require a long-term nursing facility or home care. Mortality after a hip fracture is estimated to range from 12 % to 35 %, more than that expected in the general population. The risk of a woman dying from a hip fracture (2.8 %) is equal to that of dying from breast cancer and four times greater than that for endometrial cancer (0.7 %). The highest mortality typically occurs within the first 6 months following a fracture; however, some studies show a sustained effect. Often the most serious consequences of osteoporosis are lowered self-esteem, loss of mobility, and decreased independence, together with the accompanying anxiety, depression, and loss of social activities.

Monetary costs associated with osteoporotic fractures are tremendous: about US $40 million are spent per day to treat these fractures in the USA, which adds up to US $14 billion annually for medical, hospital, and nursing home care and lost productivity. Hip fractures alone account for about 60% of these costs, and fractures at all other sites about 40%. The annual total direct hospital costs of hip fractures have been estimated at 300, 600, and 850 million euros in Sweden, France, and the UK, respectively. The total costs for osteoporotic fractures have been estimated at US $1.3 billion annually. In many countries, the population as a whole is living longer, and the proportion of old people within the population is increasing, especially those aged 85 years or more. Estimates made in 2002 indicated that in most areas of the world the frequency of hip fractures is increasing by 1.3% per year. Global demographic changes are expected to increase the incidence of hip fractures nearly fourfold by the year 2050. Each year osteoporotic fractures affect more women than heart attacks, strokes, and breast cancer combined. Indeed, the economic costs of osteoporosis are as significant as those associated with other important diseases such as chronic obstructive pulmonary disease, myocardial infarction, stroke, and breast cancer.

Therefore, it is abundantly clear that osteoporosis poses a *major public health threat* and arresting this disorder should be a primary goal of our preventive efforts in the coming century. Although osteoporosis is totally preventable, the incidence of this disorder has been increasing dramatically because the problem has not been properly addressed. With increased awareness of both the public and the medical community, osteoporosis could soon be a disease of the past, such as rickets or polio. To eliminate osteoporosis, the normal structure and function of bone must be better understood and taken into account in any future preventive and therapeutic measures.

Despite the fact that osteoporosis is one of the most extensive and costly public health problems, there is no single medical discipline that specialises in osteoporosis. Osteoporosis still falls into a kind of *"no-doctor's land."* The usual specialists available to the patients are internists, gynecologists, or endocrinologists, but none of these really specialised in osteoporosis by training. However, all physicians have a duty to provide patients with the knowledge they need to make their own informed decisions. Patients on their part have a responsibility to learn as much as they can about keeping themselves healthy and to work with their doctors to find individual strategies and solutions to

Even a small percentage reduction in the incidence of hip fractures could save several thousand lives and millions of dollars each year.

Today fewer than 10% of those who have severe osteoporosis with presence of fractures are being tested and treated!

Understanding osteoporosis is the first step to its elimination.

Don't wait and expect
action from others –
initiate it yourself!

build up and to protect the strength of their bones. The public, meanwhile, is becoming increasingly aware of osteoporosis primarily due to media interest. Many newspapers, magazines, and television news shows have begun to cover major findings in osteoporosis research because so many of their readers and viewers are affected. One recent poll showed that public awareness of the existence of osteoporosis has increased from 15 % to 85 % in the last few years. *Clinical osteology* (including osteoporosis as the most frequent condition) has now become an important and independent specialty which encompasses all aspects of bone and its disorders (including nursing, nutrition, exercise, physiology, and physical therapy). Together these form an integral part of any program designed to prevent osteoporosis and of any protocols for its treatment. Heightened awareness, closer cooperation between internists, surgeons, gynecologists, and pediatricians should lead to improved interdisciplinary care, better functional outcome, and lower national costs. A change in approach may also facilitate these goals in the future and that is: direct-to-consumer availability of densitometry and drugs for prevention of osteoporosis. This could be achieved by the establishment of consultation rooms in pharmacies or drug stores, for example; it has already been successfully started in some cities in the USA and Europe. In other words: don't rely only on doctors; take matters into your own hands. Each and every one of us is obligated to preserve his/her own skeletal structure and function throughout life. We are responsible for ourselves: "*Bone is everyBody's Business*".

Bone: An Architectural Masterpiece

The structure, function, physiology, normal processes of preservation and maintenance of the skeleton, as well as the pathologic processes underlying osteoporosis are briefly outlined in this chapter. Detailed knowledge of these processes is essential for directed research, development, and successful application of preventive and therapeutic drugs.

The skeleton consists of 220 bones and constitutes about 15 % of the total body weight. Bone has four main tasks to fulfill:

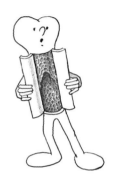

► Support and locomotion
► Protection: the skeleton protects the body from possibly harmful outside influences. For example, the ribs shelter the heart and lungs, and the cranial bones protect the brain.
► Storehouse for minerals: The skeleton is the largest depot for minerals in the body. Ninety-nine per cent of calcium, 85 % of phosphate, and 50 % of magnesium are stored in the bones. Approximately 1–1.5 kg calcium is built into the skeleton in the form of hydroxyapatite.
► Storehouse for bone matrix proteins: The mineralised bone substance consists of about 50 % organic material: 25 % matrix (ground substance) and 25 % water. The matrix contains 90 % collagen type I and 10 % other proteins such as glycoprotein, osteocalcin, osteonectin, bone sialoprotein, osteopontin, and fibronectin, as well as various proteoglycans. All these proteins are synthesised and secreted by osteoblasts and have a variety of functions, such as seeding crystal formation, binding calcium crystals, and serving as sites for attachment of bone cells. Collagen also has direct effects on important bone cell functions including apoptosis, cell proliferation

Creating healthy bones is like mixing good cement. You need the right balance of a variety of things: nutrition, exercise and genetics.

and differentiation, which are under complex control from the cell surface to the nucleus. These research findings on collagen control and function could be used as a basis to design new treatments for osteoporosis. Although collagen may have less effect on bone strength and stiffness than do minerals, it may still have a profound effect on bone fragility. Collagen changes that occur with age and reduce bone toughness may be an important factor in the risk of fracture. Bone matrix also contains proteins such as bone morphogenic proteins (BMPs), thrombospondin-2, and metalloproteinases that stimulate or inhibit the actions of bone cells. Future research in this area might be to find ways to "inhibit the inhibitors," resulting in increased bone precursors that would develop into cells that increase bone mass, that is, bone formation.

Bone has two mechanical functions to fulfill: weight-bearing and flexibility. Specific structural organisations, from the macroscopic through the microscopic to the molecular, enable bone to perform these functions:

▶ Configuration and size of bones
▶ Proportion of compact (cortical) to cancellous (trabecular) bone adapted to weight bearing
▶ Trabecular bone structure with "nodes" to support weight (a "node" comprises the junction of three or more trabeculae)
▶ Lamellar organisation of the bony tissue
▶ Degree of mineralisation of bone tissue
▶ Arrangement of collagen fibres and filaments, together with non-collagenous matrix proteins (NCPs)
▶ Cable-like organisation of collagen molecules and their "cross-linking."

Building bone up is like building a brick wall: the "cement" is composed of collagen and other matrix constituents, while crystals of calcium and phosphate constitute the mineral "bricks". Constituents of bone – perfectly balanced for maximum activity.

The elasticity of bone is achieved mainly by a special mixture of its component parts, known as "two-phase-component" in the building industry. Bone consists of the matrix (the material laid down by the osteoblasts) made up of layers of collagen molecules between which crystalline calcium and phosphate are deposited. This "passive mineralisation" leads bone gradually to become mineralised with an increasing bone mineral density as the bone gets older. The new matrix begins to mineralise after about 5–10 days from the time of deposition (*primary mineralisation*). After completion of the bone remodelling

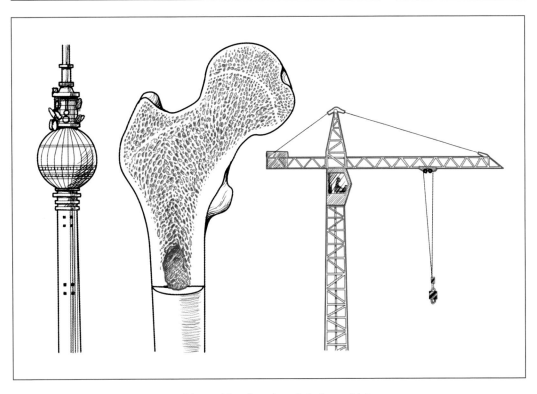

Fig. 2.1. Architectural organisation of femoral head, neck, and shaft, combining the two principles of construction for maximal weight bearing: tubular structure illustrated by the television tower and trabecular structure by the crane

cycle, a phase of *secondary mineralisation* begins. This process consists of a slow and gradual maturation of the mineral component, including an increase in the amount of crystals and/or an augmentation of crystal size toward its maximum dimension. This secondary mineralisation progressively augments the mineral content in the bone matrix. At the end of the primary mineralisation, mineral content represents only about 50% of the maximum degree of mineralisation obtained at the end of the secondary mineralisation phase. Various trace elements, water, and mucopolysaccharides serve as binding-material (glue) which binds the proteins and minerals firmly together. Collagen is responsible for the elasticity and flexibility of bone while the minerals provide strength and rigidity. The bundles of collagen fi-

Bone is rigid but flexible, hard but not brittle.

Bone mass and bone density are not synonymous – density depends also on mineralization.

bers are arranged parallel to the layers of matrix and are connected by cement lines. In adult bone, the degree of mineralisation depends on the rate of remodelling. That means that the biologic determinant of mineralisation is the rate of bone turnover. These correlations also demonstrate that "bone mass" and "bone mineral density" (BMD), often used synonymously, are two different entities. Indeed, the term "bone mineral density" has been introduced in the interpretation of the positive effects of the bisphosphonates on fracture risk.

The external aspect of bone conceals its inner architecture. The two main supporting structures of bone are only recognised in X-ray films or bone biopsy sections:

▶ *Compact, cortical bone*: It forms the outer layer of the long bones, is very densely packed and hard, and has a slow metabolic rate. Therefore, cortical bone is broken down and replaced at a much slower rate than trabecular bone. The layer of cortical bone of the long tubular bones (femur, humerus) consists of osteons or Haversian systems, which are longitudinally oriented cylinders about 5 mm long and made up of 5–20 "rings."
▶ *Spongy, cancellous, trabecular bone*, sometimes also known as ossicles: The axial skeleton (cranium, vertebral column, thorax, and pelvis) has a different and specialised construction. At first glance the trabeculae appear to be randomly distributed but closer inspection reveals that they are oriented precisely along the lines of stress and weight bearing ("trajection lines"), producing sponge-like and lattice-like structures. The more closely the trabecular "nodes" are spaced, the greater the stability and strength of the bone.

Cortical bone has three surfaces and each has different anatomic features:

▶ The *endosteal envelope*, which faces the marrow cavity and comprises a high surface area and therefore supports a high bone turnover
▶ The *periosteal envelope*, which is the outer surface of the bone to which the tendons, ligaments and muscles are attached
▶ The *intracortical envelope*, with bone surfaces inside the Haversian system, the osteons

The *skeleton* can be divided into two main compartments:

▶ *Axial skeleton*: This refers to the spine and proximal femur. The bone in this area is primarily trabecular with a high turnover.
▶ *Appendicular skeleton*: This refers to the long bones of the legs and arms. The bone in these areas is primarily cortical with a low turnover.

Approximately 80 % of bone is cortical and only 20 % is trabecular. They undergo *different rates of remodelling:*

▶ *Cortical bone* is very dense, is 90 % calcified, has a very low surface/volume ratio, and therefore has a very slow remodelling rate.
▶ In contrast, *cancellous bone* has a porous structure and a large surface area. About 25 % of cancellous bone is remodelled annually compared to only 2.5 % of cortical bone. It therefore follows that the decrease in bone is first manifest in bones with a large proportion of trabeculae and therefore with a higher surface area.

The *proportion of trabecular bone* varies in different skeletal regions:

▶ Lumbar vertebrae 75 %
▶ Heels 70 %
▶ Proximal femur 50 %–75 %
▶ Distal radius 25 %
▶ Middle of the radius <5 %

Bone: A Permanent Building and Rebuilding Site

Bone is a dynamic organ, highly vascularised, and very active metabolically. Few bones are completely developed at birth; most continue to be formed slowly out of cartilage or connective tissue, which are converted into the hard, lamellar components of the skeleton. Growth of bones ("modelling") comes to an end at puberty with ossification of the "growth plates." Modelling is of particular interest as bone is much more capable of reacting to external loads during growth than at any other time. About 90 % of adult bone is formed by the end of adolescence and subsequent gains during adulthood are very small.

Bone is a dynamic, living tissue that is constantly adapting to mechanical stress.

Table 2.1. Statistics of bone remodelling by the basic multicellular unit (BMU) in the adult. (From A. Michael Parfitt in Manolagas [A86])

Dynamic bone parameters
• 3–4 million BMUs initiated per year
• 1 million BMUs operating at any given moment
• BMU about 1–2 mm long and 0.2–0.4 mm wide
• Lifespan of BMU about 6–9 months
• Speed of BMU about 25 µm/day
• Lifespan of active osteoclasts about 2 weeks
• Lifespan of active osteoblasts about 3 months
• Interval between successive remodelling events at the same site about 2–5 years
• Rate of turnover of the whole skeleton about 10% per year*

* The 10% per year approximation for the whole skeleton is based on an average 4% turnover per year in cortical bone, which represents about 75% of the entire skeleton; and an average 28% turnover per year in trabecular bone, which represents roughly 25% of the skeleton (from S. C. Manolagas, 2000)

Wolff's law:
Putting stress on bones causes them to form more bone. And lack of stress on bones causes bone loss.

During adulthood there is a continuous process of remodelling which maintains the skeleton and adapts the bones to the changing external circumstances. Nevertheless, as the body ages, bone loses some of its strength and elasticity and therefore breaks more easily. This is due to loss of mineral and changes in the bone matrix. Bones undergo a constant process of removal and replacement so that the components of bone are exchanged at regular intervals. This process is called *remodelling* and serves the following purposes:

▶ Mobilisation of calcium in the framework of calcium homeostasis
▶ Replacement of old osseous tissue
▶ Skeletal adaptation to different loads, weight-bearing and stress
▶ Repair of damaged bone, both microscopic and macroscopic

Microfractures are not detected by standard X-rays but by special microscopic techniques in bone biopsies.

The last refers not only to repair or healing of fractures of whole bones, but also to the countless perforations or breaks of the trabeculae, the "microfractures," "microdamage," or "fatigue damage" which occur constantly and which together with the thickness of the bones determine the fracture risk. As these tiny fractures accumulate, they weaken older bones and contribute to fracture risk if not quickly and adequately repaired. This, in addition to a slightly negative bone balance over time, eventually leads to reduction in structural continuity of the trabecular network and thereby loss of strength.

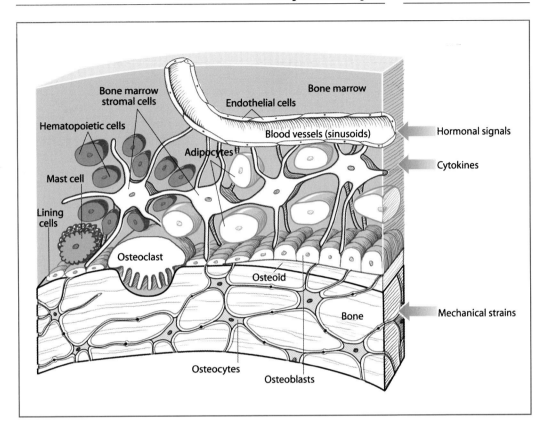

The *bone cells* constitute a specialised osseous cell system responsible for the repair, maintenance, and adaptation of bone:

▶ *Osteoclasts* ("bone breakers," "bone carvers") can resorb old, weak bone in a short period of time. These multinucleated giant cells are derived from monocytes of the bone marrow, that is, a haematopoietic cell line. The cell membrane consists of numerous "folds" – the "ruffled border" which faces the surface of the bone. The osteoclasts release quantities of proteolytic and other enzymes into the space between the ruffled membrane and the bone. These substances dissolve the minerals and some of the bone matrix; the rest is phagocytosed and metabolised in the cytoplasm of the osteoclasts. If the trabecula is thin enough, active osteoclasts may perforate and

Fig. 2.2. Interdependence of bone and marrow: together they form a single functional entity

Oestrogen is a key physiologic modulator of osteoclast formation. Its withdrawal increases osteoclast formation and this in turn leads to postmenopausal bone loss. Recent evidence indicates that oestrogen effects on bone may result from an inhibition of osteoblast apoptosis.

Osteoblasts come from the same precursor cell line as fibroblasts and adipocytes (fat cells).

Osteocytes – the watchdogs of bone. Transforming growth factor β appears to play a role in the differentiation process of the osteoblast to the osteocyte. Osteocyte apoptosis occurs at sites of microdamage, and it is proposed that dying osteocytes are targeted for removal by osteoclasts. This suggests that damaged yet viable osteocytes can send signals and can direct both osteoclastic bone resorption and osteoblastic bone formation.

transsect it, thereby disconnecting it from the trabecular network and irreversibly weakening that area of bone. Recruitment, differentiation, and activation of osteoclasts is accomplished by numerous hormones (such as parathyroid hormones, oestrogens, leptin, and thyroid hormones) as well as cytokines. Various growth factors are also involved. Recent investigations of the RANK/RANKL signalling pathway in the osteoclast have clarified mechanisms of stimulation and activation of resorption. Osteoclasts possess oestrogen receptors, by means of which oestrogen inhibits their recruitment. Androgens also act on osteoclasts. The actions of sex steroids on bone cells are discussed below.

▶ *Osteoblasts ("bone builders")* are derived from the mesenchyme in the bone marrow. They produce new bone slowly, over several weeks to replace that resorbed by the osteoclasts. Their main function is the synthesis of bone matrix, especially collagen type I but also osteocalcin, osteonectin, and bone morphogenic protein (BMP). Osteoblasts also possess receptors for oestrogen.

▶ *Osteocytes* ("bone maintainers," "bone controllers"): The osteocytes are the most numerous of all the bone cells. They develop from osteoblasts. Approximately every tenth osteoblast situated on the surface of the bone is entrapped by the newly formed bone matrix and thus becomes an osteocyte. It possesses receptors for various hormones, including PTH and sex hormones. The osteocytes occupy spaces in the bone called "lacunae" and are connected to each other and to the surface of the bone by thin channels called "canaliculi" within which long cytoplasmic processes join osteocytes to each other and thus form a circulatory system. Osteocytes possess functional gap junctions enabling them to communicate with one another (like neurons) as well as with the surface lining cells. Therefore, they are in a position to transmit the load-induced signals to preosteoblasts, which then differentiate and secrete osteoid. The total surface of combined lacunae and canaliculi has been estimated at 1,200 m². The function of osteocytes has not yet been fully elucidated, but they are known to play an important part in the transport of organic and inorganic materials within the bones. Furthermore, their strategic location enables them to function as mechanosensory cells and thus to detect the need for bone increase or decrease during functional adaptation of the skeleton, as well as the need for repair of microfractures. Osteocytes detect changes in flow of the fluid in the canaliculi and in the levels of circulating hormones such as oestrogen, glucocorticoids, and raloxifene, which influence their activities and their survival. Quite possibly they also receive impulses from the muscles, which they relay to the cells of the remodelling units at the surface of the bone. They also register the age of the bone and initiate its remodelling. On the other hand, disruption of the osteocyte network is likely to contribute to bone fragility. To summarise the function of the osteocytes: osteocytes are actively involved in remodelling and in its control mechanisms; osteocytes actively participate in ion exchange; osteocytes are mechanosensory cells, and play a major part in the functional adaptation of bone; the number (density) of osteocytes determines bone mass both for cortical and trabecular bone; decrease in osteocyte number with age is inevitably accompanied by a decrease in bone mass, as well as bone quality by impairment of repair of microfractures.

▶ *Endosteal lining cells* ("bone protectors"): these are flat cells that cover 80%–95% of the internal surface of the bones. They are presumed to develop from inactive osteoblasts. They form a protective layer and constitute a surveillance system together with osteocytes and their canaliculi. Recently, it has been shown that the endosteal lining cells may participate in activation of osteoclasts. Certain surface molecules expressed on lining cells and on osteoclast progenitors react with the receptor RANK (also found on osteoclast progenitors) and thereby set in motion a cycle of remodelling. Other important factors which participate in the remodelling cycle have also been analysed and these are: ODF (osteoclast differentiation factor), OPGL (osteoprotegerin ligand), TRANCE, and RANKL (RANK ligand). PTH, PGE_2, IL1, and 1,25 vitamin D exercise a negative influence on osteoprotegerin production and thereby stimulate resorption. Osteoblasts precursors produce M-CSF, which can activate osteoclasts. The endosteal lining cells also participate in bone remodelling. They remove fragments of bone collagen left by osteoclasts, thereby cleaning up resorption pits and initiating formation.

Lining cells were found to be intensively immunoreactive for neurokinin-2. The presence of these receptors suggests that sensory nerves may regulate the function of bone cells.

Remodelling Units

There are 2–5 million *bone remodelling units* (BRU) in the skeleton. These units, required for the maintenance and integrity of the skeleton, are of crucial importance for the development of osteoporosis.

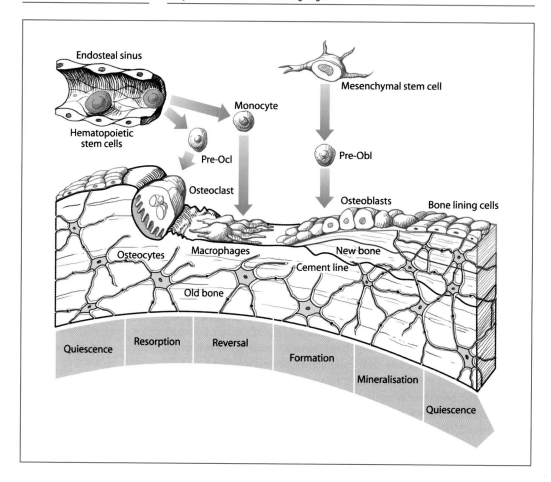

Fig. 2.3. Steps of bone remodelling in adult trabecular bone

The total quantity of bone decreases if more bone is resorbed over the years than is produced. It has been estimated that osteoporosis develops when for every 30 units of bone resorbed only 29 are produced. This negative "bone balance" has three possible causes:

▶ Increased osteoclastic activity without increased osteoblastic activity ("high turnover")
▶ Normal osteoclastic but decreased osteoblastic activity ("low turnover")
▶ Decreased osteoclastic and osteoblastic activity ("atrophy")

Table 2.2. Bone remodelling and its clinical correlations

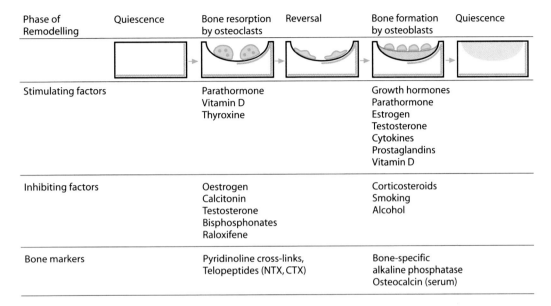

Phase of Remodelling	Quiescence	Bone resorption by osteoclasts	Reversal	Bone formation by osteoblasts	Quiescence
Stimulating factors		Parathormone Vitamin D Thyroxine		Growth hormones Parathormone Estrogen Testosterone Cytokines Prostaglandins Vitamin D	
Inhibiting factors		Oestrogen Calcitonin Testosterone Bisphosphonates Raloxifene		Corticosteroids Smoking Alcohol	
Bone markers		Pyridinoline cross-links, Telopeptides (NTX, CTX)		Bone-specific alkaline phosphatase Osteocalcin (serum)	

Consequently, a decrease in bone correlates primarily with the number of BRU and with the lack of coordination between the cells of the BRU. The level of excretion of calcium and collagen metabolites in the urine reflects the degree of resorption of bone. The process of bone remodelling is as yet incompletely understood. One *remodelling cycle* takes approximately 120 days, and it has been divided into *6 phases*:

▶ Phase of quiescence: a layer of flat lining cells covers the surface of the bone
▶ Phase of resorption: preparation of osteoclasts for resorption, osteoclasts resorb the bone, which leads to formation of lacunae or pits; osteoclasts slowly undergo apoptosis
▶ Phase of reversal: osteoblasts progenitors are attracted to the resorption pit, the surface of the resorption lacuna is prepared for new bone production by monocytes and endosteal lining cells
▶ Phase of early formation: production of osteoid by active osteoblasts
▶ Phase of late formation: mineralisation of osteoid

▶ Phase of quiescence: the active osteoblasts turn into the flat endosteal lining cells

The phase of resorption is completed within 2 weeks, while that of mineralisation may take months and depends on the presence of active metabolites of vitamin D. On completion of a remodelling cycle a *"structural bone unit"* is formed, about 35 million in the whole skeleton. Eight per cent of the skeleton is replaced annually by the activity of the bone remodelling units.

The following four *stages of osteoclast activity* are involved:

Most preventive therapies inhibits osteoclastic resorption of bone.

▶ Formation, differentiation and apoptosis of osteoclasts (RANKL)
▶ Migration and attachment on bone surface ($\alpha v \beta 3$ integrins)
▶ Acidification and solution of mineral (V-H+-ATPase, chloride channels)
▶ Dissolution of matrix (cathepsin K)

Currently, the majority of the treatments tested so far targets inhibition of bone resorption.

Control of Bone Remodelling: A Network of Complex Mechanisms

The skeleton possesses an efficient feedback-controlled system that continuously integrates signals and responses which sustain its function of delivering calcium while maintaining strength. How do osteoclasts, osteoblasts, osteocytes, and mesenchymal and haematopoietic cells cooperate to achieve such a perfect balance between resorption and formation? This complex system is just starting to be unravelled. There appear to be five groups of mechanisms regulating bone mass:

▶ *Systemic hormones*: The most important hormones are parathyroid hormone (PTH), calcitonin, thyroid hormone, insulin, growth hormone, cortisone, and sex hormones, and of these oestrogens regulate mainly osteoclastic activity and thus bone resorption. PTH, together with vitamin D, is the principal regulator of calcium homeostasis. PTH exerts its effects by way of actions on the bone cells as well as on other organs such as the kidney or the gut. On

Table 2.3. Hormonal and local regulators of bone remodelling

Hormones
Polypeptide hormones • Parathyroid hormone (PTH) • Calcitonin • Insulin • Growth hormone Steroid hormones • 1,25-Dihydroxyvitamin D3 • Glucocorticoids • Sex steroids Thyroid hormones
Local factors

Synthesised by bone cells
• IGF-I and IGF-II
• β-2-microglobulin
• TGF-β
• BMPs
• FGFs
• PDGF
Synthesised by bone-related tissue
• Cartilage-derived
  – IGF-I
  – FGFs
  – TGF-β
• Blood cell-derived
  – G-CSF
  – GM-CSF
  – IL1
  – TNF
• Other factors
  – Prostaglandins
  – Binding proteins

bone, PTH exerts its influence mainly by participation in the mechanisms controlling bone turnover. Androgens are also important in bone formation. Osteoblasts and osteocytes, as well as mononuclear and endothelial cells in the bone marrow, possess receptors for androgen; the pattern and expression of the receptors is similar in men and women. Fat cells also have receptors for sex hormones, which they are able to metabolise by means of aromatases. Signifi-

Fig. 2.4. PTH and vitamin D: control of calcium homeo-stasis. *ECF*, extracellular fluid. [Modified from Brown et al. (Endocrinologist 1994, 4:419– 426)]

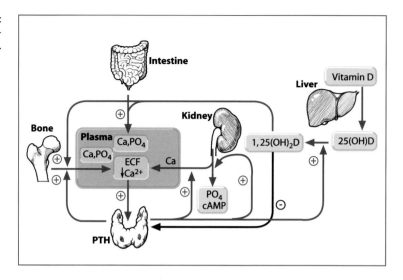

Fig. 2.4. PTH and vitamin D: control of calcium homeo-stasis. *ECF*, extracellular fluid. [Modified from Brown et al. (Endocrinologist 1994, 4:419– 426)]

Bone cells are impartial sexually: they have recep-tors for both oestrogen and testosterone, which play synergistic roles.

cant levels of both oestrogens and androgens are present in the blood in men and in women and both hormones play important, but not necessarily identical roles in bone metabolism. For exam-ple, androgens may act on osteoblasts during mineralisation, while oestrogens more likely effect osteoblasts at an earlier stage during matrix formation. Moreover, the sex hormones may also act at dif-ferent sites on the bones – for example, androgens are important in the control of periosteal bone formation, which contributes to the greater width of the cortex in men. There are receptors for oestro-gen and for testosterone on osteoblasts, osteoclasts, and osteocytes, but one or other of the sex hormones may dominate at different stages of the remodelling cycle. Androgens in particular exercise a strong influence on bone formation and resorption by way of local enzymes, cytokines, adhesion molecules, and growth factors. An-drogens increase BMD in women as well as in men, and in normal as well as in some pathologic conditions. Moreover, when given to-gether therapeutically the two hormones increase BMD more than oestrogen given alone. Other influences such as muscular mass, strength, activity, and mechanical strain may stimulate osteoana-bolic activity – that is, bone formation while inhibiting bone re-sorption. It is essential to stress that the highly complicated mech-anisms controlling bone remodelling are only briefly outlined here,

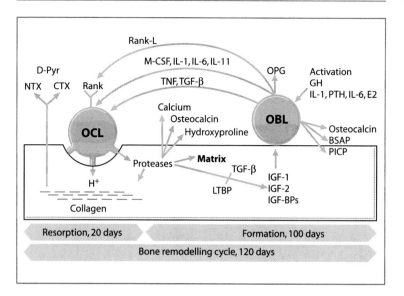

Fig. 2.5. Schematic presentation of factors controlling bone resorption and formation. *OCL*, osteoclast, *OBL*, osteoblast. The osteoblast synthesises cytokines and growth factors that activate osteoclasts. The two major ones essential for osteoclastogenesis are macrophage colony-stimulating factor (M-CSF) and osteoprotegerin ligand (OPGL), also called Rank-L. Rank-L activates its receptor Rank on the osteoclast. Osteoprotegerin (OPG) is a dummy receptor for Rank-L and can suppress osteoclastogenesis if it binds enough OPG. (Modified from Rosen and Bilzikian [A120])

but elucidation of their pathways inevitably leads to disclosure of additional points of possible therapeutic intervention.

▶ *Local cytokines and signals*: Also significant are local cytokines, electromagnetic potentials and, most importantly, signals transmitted over intercellular networks. Bone cells synthesise whole families of cytokines: for example, IGF-I, IGF-II, β_2-microglobulin, IL-1, IL-6, TGF-β, BMPs, FGFs, and PDGF. Prostaglandins play a significant part in resorption of bone during immobilisation. Another member of the tumour necrosis factor receptor family produced by osteoblasts is osteoprotegerin (OPG), which blocks osteoclast differentiation from precursor cells und so prevents resorption. In fact, OPG could represent the long sought-after molecular link between arterial calcification and bone resorption, which underlies the clinical coincidence of vascular disease and osteoporosis most

Systemic, central orders to bone, such as circulating hormones, are translated into specific local instructions – and there are many pathways for these to travel along.

prevalent in postmenopausal women and elderly people. OPG could represent a novel pathway for possible manipulation of bone remodelling.

Vitamin D: when the sun is obscured, take a tablet instead.

▶ *Vitamins and minerals*: The bone cells as well as the surrounding cell systems are also influenced by various vitamins, minerals, and other factors. Vitamin D, K, C, B_6, and A are all required for the normal metabolism of collagen and for mineralisation of osteoid.

Mechanical loading: builds bone mass in childhood, maintains it in adults.

▶ *Mechanical loading*: Exercise may improve bone mass and bone strength in children and adolescents. However, the osteogenic potential diminishes at the end of puberty and longitudinal growth of the bones. The adult skeleton is only moderately responsive to mechanical loading. A new way which might be useful to manipulate bone tissue is high-frequency, low-amplitude "vibration" exercise, combined with rest periods between loading events. Bone tissue cells must transduce an extracellular mechanical signal into an intracellular response. A mechanoreceptor is known to be a structure made up of extracellular and intracellular proteins linked to transmembrane channels. Touch sensation, proprioception and blood pressure regulation are mediated by ion channels. It has been proposed that osteocyte processes are tethered to the extracellular matrix and that these tethers amplify cell membrane strains. Presumably, extracellular fluid flow creates drag on the tethers, thus stretching the cell membrane.

Various genes and transcription factors still require elucidation.

▶ *Transcriptional regulation and genes*: There exist a number of transcriptional factors that control osteogenesis and differentiation of osteoblasts. These include runt-related transcription factor 2 (Runx2), Osterix (Osx), and sex determining region Y-box 9 (Sox9), "master" regulators of osteogenesis. Also, new genes responsible for hereditary skeletal disorders could provide new therapeutic opportunities. For example, the identification of LRP5 as a key molecule in bone regulation was shown recently to promote osteoblastic differentiation.

Leptin: Role of the Central Nervous System in Regulation of Bone

The observation that overweight individuals are less susceptible to osteoporosis hints at a link between obesity and the skeleton. It was first suggested that the effects of increased weight-bearing might protect

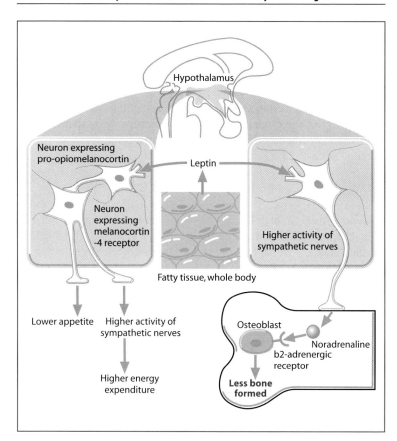

Fig. 2.6. Central nervous participation via leptin in bone turnover. (Modified from Harada and Rodan [A61])

bone mass. However, experimental studies have implicated leptin: a hormone produced by fat cells which interacts with neurons in the brain and thereby influences weight. It was then discovered that in mice leptin is also antiosteogenic and it was speculated that increased bone mass in obese people may result from resistance to leptin's antiosteogenic activity. Leptin is released into the bloodstream in proportion to the amount of body fat. It regulates the body's energy balance and bone mass by binding to certain receptor proteins of specific neurons in the hypothalamus of the brain, which in turn activate sympathetic nerves. These extend into the bone, where they stimulate release of the neurotransmitter noradrenaline, which then stimulates β2-adrenergic receptors on osteoblasts, inhibiting osteoblastic activity. Leptin inhibits bone formation through its action on already differentiated osteoblasts and has no overt effect on osteoclast differentiation or function. These results seem to suggest that the millions of patients who have been treated with "β blockers" such as propranolol for hypertension should have increased bone mass – an argument for reassessing these clinical studies with respect to changes in bone density. The identification of leptin as a powerful inhibitor of bone formation definitely has potential therapeutic implications in the future.

Peak Bone Mass: An Investment for a Healthier Life

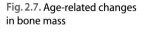

Peak bone mass is a strong predictor of later osteoporotic fractures. When we are born, our skeleton contains approximately 25 g of calcium. At age 30, when our bone mass reaches its peak, our skeleton harbours about 1,000 g of calcium. The risk of developing osteoporosis depends on how much bone an individual has as a young adult ("peak bone mass") and how quickly she/he loses it later in life.

The skeleton acquires the maximal bone density – "*peak bone mass*" – at 25–30 years. Thereafter at about 30 years, a negative bone balance sets in, so that on average 1 % of bone is lost every year, independent of sex. Measurements of trabecular bone density between ages 20 and 80 have shown reductions of approximately 50 % in density. This bone loss is apparently genetically programmed. Therefore, the bones are like a bank savings account for calcium. If the calcium supply is adequate, savings deposits are made and the calcium bone bank accounts builds up. If the dietary calcium intake is too low, then withdrawals of calcium are made from the skeleton.

Calcium tends to be stored in the bone tissue during the day and slowly released during the night. A bone biopsy study has shown that the loss of bone occurs fairly equally in all regions of the skeleton, per-

Fig. 2.7. Age-related changes in bone mass

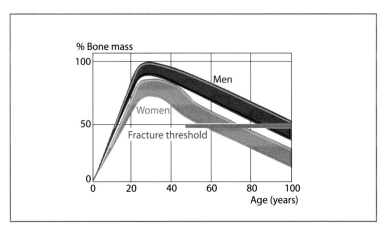

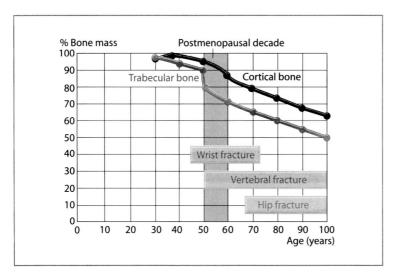

Fig. 2.8. Correlation between predominant trabecular bone loss and incidence of types of fractures

haps slightly more in the vertebral bodies and the proximal femur. In postmenopausal women, the decline in oestrogen is accompanied by an increase of bone loss of up to 4% annually. This implies that women may lose 40% of their bone mass from age 40 to 70 years. During the same period men lose only about 12%.

The goal of any bone-building programme is two-fold: Maximise genetic peak bone mass and minimise bone loss!

Osteoporosis: How to Define it

First What It Is Not

The most common myths and misconceptions about osteoporosis:

- I am too young to get osteoporosis.
- Only women get osteoporosis.
- I drink lots of milk and therefore I won't get osteoporosis.
- My mother had osteoporosis and so I am doomed to have it too.
- I will know when I get it.

► Just thin bones
► A normal, unavoidable part of the aging process
► Common all over the world
► A inevitable disorder of postmenopausal women and all elderly people

Definitions of Osteoporosis

The word osteoporosis literally means porous bone, that is, bone density is low and the bones are thin. But bone does not fracture due to thinness alone. The World Health Organisation (WHO) defines *osteoporosis* as

> "a systemic skeletal disorder characterised by a low bone mass and microarchitectural deterioration of bone tissue, with a subsequent increase in bone fragility and susceptibility to fracture."

The first Consensus Conference on Osteoporosis of the new millennium proposed a new definition of osteoporosis as

> "a skeletal disorder characterised by compromised bone strength predisposing to an increased risk of fracture."

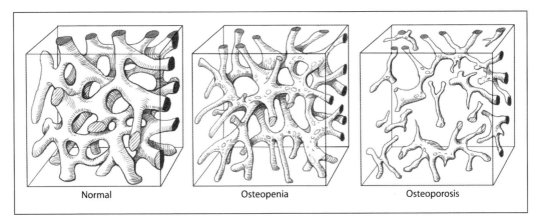

Fig. 3.1. Progressive architectural deterioration of cancellous bone: increased osteoclastic resorption cavities and marked attenuation of cancellous bone (osteopenia); disconnected trabeculae, no longer a network (established osteoporosis)

However, in order to better understand the etiology of osteoporotic fractures and the effects of therapy on fracture risk, it is essential to recognise the factors that govern bone strength. The strength of an individual bone (and of the whole skeleton) depends on its mass, shape, and the quality of the bone itself.

Numerous large studies have already confirmed the connection between bone density, strength, and fracture risk. Density is responsible for 60%–90% of the strength of bone. From the outside however, osteoporotic bones may have the same size and may even look like normal bones, but inside they are brittle, with thin cortical bone and a loss of trabeculae.

Osteoporosis is largely a disease of modern civilisation.

Low bone mass has proved to be the most important objective predictor of fracture risk. The lower the bone mass, the weaker the bone and the less force required to cause a fracture. Therefore, according to the WHO (The WHO Study Group 1994) osteoporosis in postmenopausal women has also been defined in terms of bone density measurement and based on a comparison of the patients' measurement to peak adult bone mass (PABM) as follows:

"Osteoporosis is present when the bone mass is more than 2.5 standard deviations (SD) below that of healthy premenopausal adult females, the T-score."

The hip and/or the lumbar spine are measured by the DXA-method to obtain the T-score. The cutoff point of 2.5 SD below PABM is based on epidemiological data derived from a population of postmenopausal white women, 50% of whom had already suffered a fragility fracture. These criteria of the WHO were not meant to be applied to healthy, oestrogen-replete premenopausal women, women of other races, young men, or children. Nevertheless, low bone mass in any individual is still the most important factor in the determination of fragility fractures.

> Osteopenia has been defined by a T-score <−1.0 and −2.5.

Osteopenia in any body is the clarion call: the warning signal for immediate preventive therapy.

As the emphasis on skeletal health shifts from treatment to prevention, the diagnostic term of osteopenia may take on increasing importance, especially in combination with the evaluation of the major risk factors. Hence, postmenopausal women with osteopenia should be targeted for prevention strategies to preserve their skeletal mass. Patients with osteopenia and relevant risk factors should be treated early with effective drugs to prevent fragility fractures.

Osteoporosis: Which Bones Are Vulnerable

The greater the surface area for remodelling, the more vulnerable the bone.

Low bone density is an even better predictor of fracture risk than increased cholesterol is of having a heart attack or high blood pressure is of having a stroke.

Where and how does bone resorption occur? The bone cells carry out their remodelling preferably on the inner surface of bone, the endosteum. Bones with a large component of cancellous bone present the largest surface area to bone cells for remodelling: these bones include the vertebral bodies, the femoral neck, the ribs, the wrist, and the heel. Due to their immense surface, these cancellous bones are resorbed five times as fast as the cortical bone of the long bones. Considered sequentially, the ossicles in the middle of the bone disappear first, especially those at the horizontal "stress" lines. The vertical "pillars," which carry greater loads, remain intact for longer periods and are seen as vertical stripes on X-ray. In vitro and in vivo studies have shown that bone density is indeed responsible for 50%–80% of the strength of bone and therefore constitutes a very important risk factor, particularly in postmenopausal women. As numerous prospective studies have demonstrated, the risk of a fracture increases exponentially with the decrease in density: a reduction of 10%–15% in bone density doubles the fracture risk.

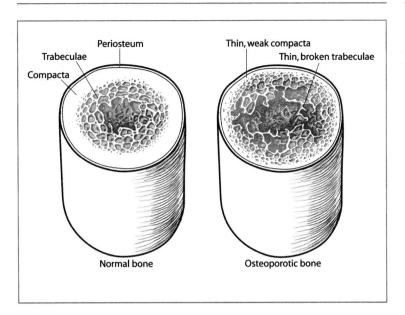

Fig. 3.2. Osteoporotic tubular bone: shrinkage of cortical width; rarefaction and discontinuity of trabecular network

In the figure:
- Compacta
- Trabeculae
- Periosteum
- Thin, weak compacta
- Thin, broken trabeculae
- Normal bone
- Osteoporotic bone

Osteoporosis: Also a Question of Quality

Bone does not break only because it is thin – as indicated by the fact that half of all people with decreased bone density never sustain a fracture. The recognition that osteoporosis is far more complex than previously thought suggests that factors in addition to bone mineral density may contribute to bone fragility and therapeutic effectiveness. Recent studies have shown that osteoporosis is also a question of the quality of bone. Perforations, that is, "microfractures" of trabeculae occur constantly throughout life and normal activity, and these lead to a decrease in bone strength and weight-bearing ability – and of course require immediate repair. Moreover, previous thinning of the trabeculae because of decreased osteoblastic activity accelerates the destruction of the microarchitecture. Disconnected trabeculae are functionally useless and are rapidly resorbed. Should a situation arise in which numerous microfractures are not completely repaired, a critical point will eventually be reached at which the bone will break. Should the bone structure be qualitatively inferior to begin with, bones of even normal thickness may break. This is an important point to take into account and has already been demonstrated in osteoporosis in hypo-

Bone cells detect damage, resorb old bone and replace it with new bone: the bone remodelling process. Inadequate repair of microfractures reduces the quality of bone.

gonadal men. Studies on mineral density by magnetic resonance microradiography have shown a marked deterioration in microarchitecture in the spine and hips of these patients – more than would be expected from the results of densitometry. An important (even crucial) aim of osteoanabolic therapy is to re-establish the microarchitecture. This goal could probably be achieved in the not-too-distant future by a combination of drugs: administration of basic fibroblast growth factor, which induces formation of new trabeculae and promotes restoration of connectivity, both of which could be maintained by antiresorptive agents and/or PTH. These results have been achieved in osteoporotic animal models. Trials in humans have not yet been published.

Generally speaking, osteoporotic fractures are caused by *8 different abnormalities of bone:*

▶ Reduced thickness (density)
▶ Unequal proportions of compact and cancellous bone
▶ Decrease in number of "knots" in the cancellous bone
▶ Transsection of trabeculae caused by osteoclasts
▶ Inadequate bone formation
▶ Inadequate mineralisation of bone matrix (osteoid)
▶ Anomalies of structure and binding of collagen molecules ("crosslinking")
▶ Faulty repair mechanisms

Fastest way to reduce fragility: inhibit resorption and maintain mineralisation by vitamin D and calcium.

How can fragility be reduced? There are *two ways to make bones stronger:*

▶ Increase bone mineral density and distribute bone mass more effectively, i. e., increase bone tissue where the mechanical demands are greatest ("extrinsic biomechanical properties")
▶ Improve the material properties of bone tissue, from the microscopic to the molecular level ("intrinsic biochemical properties")

An effective treatment for bone fragility should improve the extrinsic biomechanical properties of bone but at the same time not substantially impair the intrinsic properties. Strong inhibitors of bone resorption such as bisphosphonates can reduce bone turnover by 80 %–90 %, causing a gain in bone mineral density. Due to reduced bone remodelling, the mean tissue age of bone is increased, as is bone mineralisation. Properly mineralised bone has the best combination of stiffness and brittleness, while poorly mineralised bone tends to be very weak with increased displacement, and hypermineralised bone is too brittle with decreased displacement. Consequently, in treating osteoporosis attention must be paid to bone density, to improvement of the microarchitecture, to mineralisation, and to the repair mechanisms. Today, with the modern bisphosphonates, it is no longer a problem to fill up resorption lacunae, to increase mineralisation, and to thicken attenuated trabeculae. At present, there is no evidence that microdamage accumulation occurs under treatment with bisphosphonates. However, it is not yet possible – as far as we know from experimental studies – to restore the trabecular network or the shape of bone that has been destroyed. The basic anatomic and structural properties of bone influence the load-carrying capacity and the changes in osteoporosis determine the fracture risk. New methods are needed to provide insight into the causes of bone fragility and the effects of drug therapies.

How to Define "Fracture"? Not So Simple!

A fracture has been defined as an "acute discontinuity" in a bone. When there does not appear to be adequate trauma, the terms "pathologic fracture," "fragility fracture," or "low trauma fracture" are used, and these of course need clarification. "Fatigue fractures" develop slowly – a summation of numerous microfractures which were not properly repaired. Examples are fatigue fractures of the metatarsals in marathon runners or fractures of the pelvic girdle in patients with age-related osteoporosis. These microfractures should not be confused with "Looser's zones" in patients with osteomalacia (rickets). "Infractions" are partial fractures of the long bones when a localised unilateral break of the cortex occurs. "Vertebral compression fractures" often occur in stages and initially remain undetected until a total collapse of the vertebral body has taken place.

Osteoporosis causes symptoms only if a fracture has occurred.

Vertebral (Spinal) Fractures

As mentioned above, a vertebral fracture rarely occurs in osteoporosis because of sudden trauma but rather in stages as a result of numerous microfractures. Moderate decrease in height of the vertebral bodies

Fig. 3.3. Effects of progressive compression fractures in the vertebrae

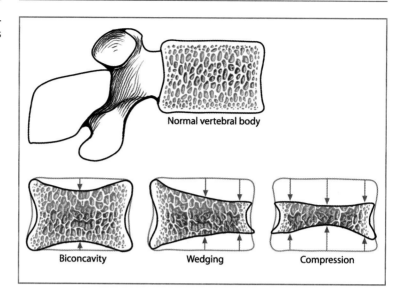

can only be detected by sequential films. Three grades of vertebral deformities are recognised:

▶ End-plate deformity
▶ Anterior wedge deformity
▶ Compression deformity

Biconcave deformities, with depression of the upper and lower cortices of the vertebral bodies are the first to appear. Occasionally, focal depression may be caused by material from an intervertebral disk (Schmorl's knots). Fractures of the vertebral bodies have been named according to the shape of the deformity:

▶ Endplate fracture
▶ Anterior wedging
▶ Posterior wedging
▶ Compression (crush)

The last type involves the whole vertebral body. The deformity grading system in use comprises 6 degrees of severity and is based on a percentage reduction in vertebral height. Other types of deformities

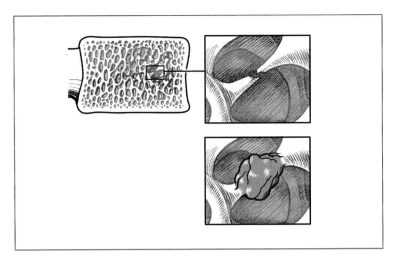

Fig. 3.4. Osteoclastic perforation of a horizontal trabecula (*upper right*) of the vertebral body (*left*), and formation of microcallus (early healing microfracture) (*lower right*)

with various grades of severity also occur. An exact definition of vertebral body fractures has great practical significance because the number and extent of such fractures are used as significant parameters in therapeutic trials. Comparison and meta-analyses of trials depend on a clear and reproducible definition of "fracture."

Hip Fractures

There are good correlations between fracture rates and the result of DXA measurements of the femoral neck, Ward's triangle and the trochanter. *Three X-ray parameters* have prognostic significance:

Ninety percent of all hip fractures among elderly women are attributed to low bone mass.

▶ Singh index
▶ Femoral neck length
▶ Femoral neck width

The *Singh index* recognises 7 trabecular groups in the proximal femur which indicate pressure or traction according to their orientation. Between them lies an area which is relatively poor in ossicles called

Up to 20% of all hip fractures are attributed to smoking.

Ward's triangle. As osteoporosis progresses, the seven groups of trabeculae are steadily resorbed, so that *three types of fractures* may result:

► Medial
► Lateral
► Intertrochanteric

Wrist Fractures

Fractures of the distal radius (Colles' fractures) occur most commonly in women between 45 and 65 years of age. These are nearly always caused by a direct fall forwards onto the outstretched arm, with distal dislocation of the hand.

Other Fractures

Other fractures associated with osteoporosis include those of the proximal humerus, the pelvis, the distal tibia, the heel, the ankle, the clavicle, and the ribs. All these bones contain a large amount of cancellous bone. In contrast, bones with a high content of cortical, compact bone such as the metatarsals, the phalanges, and the proximal radius rarely fracture.

CHAPTER 4 Subgroups of Osteoporosis: From Different Points of View

According to Spread

Osteoporosis may be *localised* to one or more skeletal regions i.e., focal or regional osteoporosis, as distinct from the classic *generalised* osteoporosis (systemic, global). The most important causative factors responsible for local bone loss are:

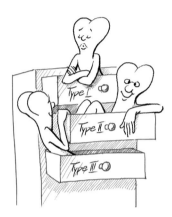

▶ *Inactivity* (immobilisation osteoporosis): The classical example is the regional osteoporosis which occurs when an extremity is immobilised either because of a fracture or a motor-neuron injury. The lack of use and movement results in increased osteoclastic resorption which, if sufficiently extensive, is also accompanied by hypercalciuria and hyperphosphaturia. On cessation of immobilisation and resumption of activity the process can be reversed and the bones normalised, especially those of children and young people.
▶ *Complex Regional Pain Syndrome* (CRPS, Sudeck's disease, algodystrophy, sympathetic reflex dystrophy): This effects mainly the hands, knees, and ankles and is characterised by swelling, pain, hyperaesthesias, and vasomotor reactions. This condition is dealt with extensively in Chap. 23.
▶ *Transient (transitory) osteoporosis*: Transient osteoporosis is a regional process first described in the pelvic bones in pregnant women. Since then, it has also been observed in knee and ankle joints in both young men and young women. The pain appears to start spontaneously without apparent prior trauma. The diagnosis is established by means of magnetic resonance imaging (MRI), which shows extensive edema of the bone marrow around the painful joint. Clinically, the process is self-limiting with complete restitution within a year.

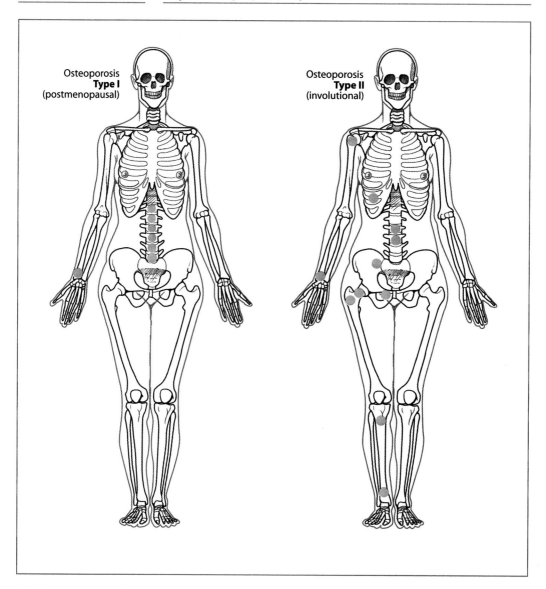

Fig. 4.1. Topographic differences in skeletal involvement between type I and type II osteoporosis

▶ *Gorham-Stout Syndrome* ("vanishing bone disease"): The cause of this rare bone disease has not yet been elucidated, though a vascular and lymphatic connection has been suggested, mainly by way of activated endothelium. It begins with osteoclastic resorption of a bone and spreads to adjoining bones. Progression is variable. Severe or life-threatening complications may occur when bones of the thorax or the vertebrae are involved. So far, the only effective therapy is administration of bisphophonates as early as possible to prevent extensive loss of bone (see Chap. 23).

▶ *Other osteolytic syndromes*: These may be due to a variety of different causes, including infections, tumours, and trauma as well as metabolic, vascular, congenital, and genetic aberrations.

▶ *Generalised (systemic) osteoporosis*: This is far more frequent than localised osteoporosis. In spite of its name, generalised osteoporosis is rarely manifest in the whole skeleton, but it does have a symmetrical distribution. Juvenile and postmenopausal osteoporoses generally effect the axial skeleton, while the age-related form also attacks the tubular bones, especially in men. Consequently, presence of a normal bone density in bones of the extremities does not rule out osteoporosis (possibly even severe) of the axial skeleton.

Rare osteoporotic and osteolytic syndromes require special consideration.

According to Sex and Age

▶ *Idiopathic juvenile osteoporosis*: This is a rare self-limiting disease of prepubertal children, usually occurring between 8 and 14 years of age. It generally manifests as compression fractures of the vertebrae accompanied by severe back pain. The differential diagnosis includes osteogenesis imperfecta, Cushing syndrome, and diseases of the bone marrow, which are diagnosed by means of peripheral blood and bone biopsy.

▶ *Idiopathic osteoporosis of young adults*: This affects primarily men between the ages of 30 and 50 years, and it is also characterised by fractures of the vertebral bodies. Biochemical parameters and bone biopsy findings show increased resorption of bone. Frequently the patients are heavy smokers, which has been implicated as a possible contributory factor. A mild form of osteogenesis imperfecta must be excluded in these patients.

▶ *Postmenopausal (type I) osteoporosis*: This is the most common form of osteoporosis and it occurs in women between 51 and 75

Postmenopausal women, and men about 10 years later, are particularly prone to bone loss.

years of age as a consequence of cessation of ovarian function. The loss of bone actually starts years beforehand and increases at the time of menopause (perimenopausal). About 30 % of all women develop osteoporosis after menopause. Cessation of oestrogen secretion leads to a decrease in IL-6 and other cytokines, which in turn leads to increased recruitment and activation of osteoclasts. In addition, bone becomes more sensitive to the resorption stimulating action of parathyroid hormones. As a consequence there is increased resorption of cancellous bone in the vertebrae and in the hip bones, with a corresponding increase in risk of fractures. Obviously, this postmenopausal form of osteoporosis occurs only in women, but men are also subject to increased bone resorption as a consequence of testosterone deficiency, though at a later stage in life.

▶ *Involutional (age-related, type II) osteoporosis*: Postmenopausal osteoporosis merges imperceptibly into the age-related type which represents part of the aging process and includes increased osteoclastic activity. A study of bone biopsies taken from normal individuals (i.e., without any known metabolic, endocrine, or osseous disorders) of different age groups has shown that the number of osteoclasts and osteoblasts increases from the age of 50 years. This indicates that bone, far from being a slow, inactive, and atrophic tissue in the older age groups, presents the picture of increased osseous remodelling. Other causative factors for involutional osteoporosis are: decreased mobility, defective vitamin D metabolism, insufficient calcium, and mild secondary hyperparathyroidism. Osteoporosis type II develops after 70 years of age and is now only twice as frequent in women as in men (however they are catching up!). Cortical bone, especially that of the femoral neck, the radius, and pelvic bones, is then also involved. About 80 % of all osteoporotic fractures occur at this time i.e., after 70 years. The arbitrary separation of these osteoporoses – type I and type II – at this stage of the patients' lives (>70 years) is of little (if any) practical value.

According to Extent

In daily clinical practice the *degree of severity* of a bone disorder must be accurately determined before decisions are made on urgency and strategy of therapy. In women, osteoporosis can be diagnosed if the bone mineral density (BMD) is 2.5 SD below the mean of a young reference population. Kanis and coworkers commented on this definition and gave diagnostic categories that may be applied to white women:

▶ *Normal bone*: a BMD value less than 1 SD below the young adult mean value
▶ *Osteopenia (borderline)*: a BMD value between 1 and 2.5 SD below the young adult mean value
▶ *Preclinical osteoporosis*: a BMD value more than 2.5 SD below the young adult mean value
▶ *Severe (manifest, established) osteoporosis*: a BMD value more than 2.5 SD below the young adult mean value in the presence of one or more fragility fractures

This definition uses the T-score as a diagnostic measure as it has already long been used in bone densitometry. Bone density results are compared to those of age-, sex-, and race-matched controls.

Remember: no single site represents the whole skeleton!

A clinical grading of osteoporosis based on measurements of bone density and the clinical picture was proposed by Minne in 1995:

▶ *Grade 0*: T-score between –1 and –2.5 SD, no fractures. This corresponds to osteopenia (as above) or also called "borderline osteoporosis." These patients are in no urgent need of therapy, which can be given without haste and monitored by bone density measurements. Generally speaking, years may elapse before fractures occur in this group in the absence of preventive therapy and of accelerated progression for whatever reason.
▶ *Grade 1*: The bone density is clearly reduced: T-score below –2.5 SD; fractures have not yet occurred, but could do so at any time. There is no time to lose and effective therapy should be administered immediately – an aminobisphosphonate is the drug of choice.
▶ *Grade 2*: T-score below –2.5 SD and vertebral fractures have already occurred. The risk of additional fractures has increased and is high. Immediate therapy continued for 1–2 years is required till the risk

has been significantly reduced. Pain relief and rehabilitation become increasingly important.

The T-score is the internationally accepted criterion for evaluation of results of clinical trials.

▶ *Grade 3*: T-score below 2.5 SD and several fractures have already occurred. Not only the vertebrae, but also other parts of the skeleton are involved such as the pelvis, the hip joint, or the arm. Pain relief and rehabilitation are essential, but antiresorptive medication is also necessary, at the very least to prevent further loss of bone.

According to Histology

Histology provides direct estimation of bone quantity, quality, mineralisation and turnover.

The trabecular bone volume in iliac crest biopsies of normal adults comprises about 20–25 vol% of the biopsy section. When this value drops to 16%, "rarefaction" of the trabeculae has occurred. Other histological parameters are also evaluated:

▶ Cortical thickness and cortical porosity
▶ Disruption of trabecular network
▶ Trabecular width. Type A = long and thin, type B = short and stout
▶ Quantity and distribution of osteoid (degree of mineralisation)
▶ Quantity and distribution of fat cells (atrophy in the endosteal region)
▶ Changes of the stromal elements (inflammatory reactions)
▶ Quantity and maturation of the haematopoietic cell lines
▶ Presence of foreign or malignant cells.

When the trabeculae are surrounded by fat cells or layers of fatty tissue, then osseous remodelling is decreased and osteoid seams are absent (bone atrophy). This particular distribution of fat cells is a sign of incipient osteoporosis, the "low turnover" type as demonstrated in sequential biopsies. Recent research has demonstrated that there is indeed a connection between fat cells and osteoblastic activity.

Histology is essential for identification of osteomalacia.

The volume, extent, and width of osteoid seams are always noted in order to estimate the presence and degree of osteomalacia. These data are required for estimating the therapeutic amounts of vitamin D required. The value for osteoid should not exceed 2 vol%. However, in older patients values of 2–5 vol% are frequently found, which indicate the presence of an "osteoporomalacia," when a low trabecular vol% is also present. A *histologic diagnosis of osteomalacia* is based on three criteria:

▶ Periosteocytic demineralisation (an early sign!)
▶ Osteoid occupies more than 50 % of the trabecular surface
▶ Width of osteoid seams more than 10 % of the total trabecular volume (vol %)

The *clinical diagnosis of osteomalacia* requires X-ray (Looser's zones), serologic investigation and evidence of a basic disorder (usually of gastrointestinal or renal origin).

Immunohistochemical evidence of bisphosphonates in bone biopsy sections is of particular interest. A comprehensive description of the significance of bone biopsies in internal medicine can be found in the atlas "Biopsy of Bone in Internal Medicine" (Bartl and Frisch 1993). Moreover, with the introduction of improved biopsy needles and the latest immunohistological techniques as well as increasing interest in bone and its cells, bone biopsies will also acquire greater significance in the investigation of disorders of bone including osteoporoses, especially secondary and drug-induced.

Histology and immuno-histology: detection of causes of secondary osteoporoses.

Osteoporosis does not choose its victims at random. We have to acknowledge that certain risk factors cannot be changed and must be accepted. But there are crucial risk factors that can and must be avoided!

Until recently, the diagnosis of osteoporosis was made only when the patient presented with painful fractures. Today, with a greater consciousness of health and healthy living we realise that recognition and avoidance of risk factors can prevent many chronic illnesses. A 50-year-old-postmenopausal woman who goes to her physician for a yearly "checkup" expects to have her blood pressure taken, her cholesterol measured, and a mammography performed – that is good medical practice. Likewise, she should ask for a bone mineral density measurement to investigate her risk for developing osteoporosis. Research even suggests that low bone mass density is a better predictor of fracture risk than increased cholesterol is of having a heart attack and high blood pressure of having a stroke. We are now aware of many genetic and acquired factors which are responsible for and/or contribute to the development of osteoporoses. Furthermore, a low bone mineral density is associated with a lower risk of breast cancer: stimulating effects of oestrogen on both trabecular bone and mammary cells may be responsible for this correlation. Another study has shown that bone density changes might be related to the progression of atherosclerosis, or vice versa, in hemodialysis patients.

Risk Factors Which Cannot (Yet) Be Influenced

Risks you can't avoid!

Genetics. The saying "as mother so daughter" applies especially to osteoporosis. A family history of an osteoporotic fracture in a first-degree relative is a powerful indicator that genetic factors may play a role in the development of osteoporosis. We know that the "peak bone mass" and the subsequent later loss of bone are genetically programmed. Studies of twins have shown that genetic factors account for up to 80% of the variance in bone mineral density, the best known

Table 5.1. Genetic syndromes featuring osteoporosis

Syndrome	Clinical features
Turner (XO)	Short stature, primary amenorrhoe
Klinefelter (XXY)	Tall stature, gynecoid features
Osteogenesis imperfecta	Blue sclerae, dental abnormalities
Ehlers-Danlos	Joint hypermobility, dislocations
Cutis laxa	Lax skin, premature aged appearance
Marfan	Tall stature, lens dislocation, aortic root dilation, "Floppy valve syndrome"
Homocystinuria	Tall stature, thrombosis, lens dislocation
Cleidocranial dysplasia	Sloped shoulders, dental abnormalities
Osteoporosis-pseudoglioma	Poor vision, early fractures
Werner	Short stature, premature aging
Hereditary sensory neuropathies	Insensitivity to pain

predictor of the risk of osteoporosis. Some loci, such as for vitamin D and oestrogen receptor genes as well as the collagen type Ia1 locus, are promising genetic determinants of bone mass, but the molecular basis of osteoporosis still remains largely undefined. Experts have also implicated gene-gene and gene-environment interactions as significant determinants of bone density and risk of osteoporosis. As yet there are no tests available to evaluate the genetic risk of osteoporosis. Nevertheless, a proper diet and exercise in childhood and youth can go a long way to ensure a peak bone mass in adulthood. Part of the heterogeneity of osteoporosis may be due to the presence of osteoporosis in a number of genetic syndromes ("syndromic osteoporosis"). Information derived from genetic studies is being used to developed markers for assessment of fracture risk and new drugs for osteoporosis. Genetic syndromes causing osteoporosis can be distinguished by careful physical examination (e.g., stature, as well as abnormalities of teeth, skin, and eyes). These features are common to a number of the syndromes listed in Table 5.1.

Peak bone mass is largely determined by genetics, which accounts for over half of the variance, but other modifiable lifestyle factors also play a role.

Race. Caucasians tend to have the lowest bone mass, and hip fractures are far more common among whites than nonwhites. Age-adjusted hip

Osteoporosis discriminates
in favour of people of colour!

Appropriate lifestyle
programmes, nutrition and
physical exercise are
essential for both sexes
and at all ages.

fracture incidence rates are higher among Scandinavian residents than other comparable populations. Afro-American women tend to have the highest bone density and lose bone less rapidly as they age.

Sex and age. Between 30 and 35 years of age osseous remodelling, i.e., resorption and formation are balanced. Thereafter the genetically determined bone loss sets in, somewhat greater in women than in men. We tend to lose bone mass at a rate of 0.5%–1% per year after the age of 30. With the onset of menopause and the drop in oestrogen secretion, the rate of osteoporosis and of fractures in women increases steadily. In men, the risk of fractures increases steadily after 75 years and then rises to over 30%. The risk increases even more dramatically with each decade of increasing age. The elderly also have an increased tendency to fall: one-third of individuals over 65 years of age will fall at least once a year. About 6% of falls for individuals over age 75 result in a fracture. Further risks of developing osteoporosis are: increasing occurrence of additional illnesses, need for various medications, deficiencies of calcium and vitamin D, decrease of physical activities, and decrease of osteoblastic activity.

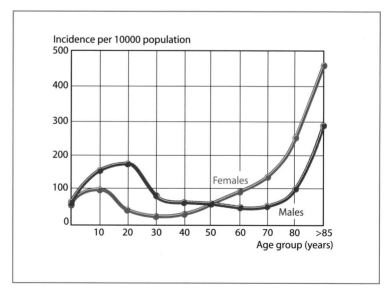

Fig. 5.1. Incidence of fractures according to sex and age. Notice time lag of about 10 years in elderly men

Previous fractures. Even if the cause is unknown, the risk of sustaining another fracture is doubled when one has already occurred. Possibly individuals with one fracture tend to fall and develop subsequent fractures at a greater rate than individuals with no history of fractures. It has been estimated that a single spontaneous vertebral fracture raises the risk of further vertebral fractures by a factor of 5, while two or more fractures increase the risk by a factor of 12.

Once bitten – twice shy! Institute immediate measures to prevent recurrence.

Pregnancy and lactation. A woman nursing a baby secretes about 500 mg calcium daily into the milk. After nursing five babies, she will have secreted some 300 g of calcium – about a third of the amount of bound calcium incorporated in the skeleton. To some extent the high levels of sex hormones during pregnancy stimulate a greater absorption of calcium from the gastrointestinal tract and a greater uptake by the bones. However, there are additional risks for osteoporosis when several weeks' bed rest is required and also if muscle relaxants and sedation are administered during pregnancy. In some cases corticosteroids are also given. In these circumstances a massive excretion of calcium and loss of bone is the inevitable result, and the pregnant women must be given calcium and vitamin D to compensate for the loss. In general, there is a decrease in bone density during pregnancy and breast-feeding, but it returns to normal after birth and weaning. Only a few women suffer fractures during this temporary decrease in bone mass.

Reproductive period: help maintain bones by supplements before, during and after.

Risk Factors Which Can Be Influenced

Chronic inactivity. Insufficient physical movement is the single most important risk factor for osteoporosis. This applies also to younger, bed-ridden patients who may loose up to 30 % of their bone mass in a few months, but may require years to regain their original bone density. When an arm is immobilised in plaster for 3 weeks because of a wrist fracture, the bones involved lose 6 % of their density. A study of bed-rest showed that trabecular bone was lost at the rate of about 1 % per week! It has been suggested that trabecular bone returns at about 1 % per month, so that restoration of bone mass is much slower than bone loss.

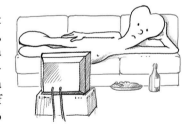

Things you *can* change!

Examples of immobilisation with rapid bone loss are:

▶ Paralysis after spinal injuries
▶ Hemiplegia after cerebrovascular events
▶ Paraplegia of the lower half of the body
▶ Immobilisation after fractures of the lower extremities in children
▶ Weightlessness in astronauts

Osteoporosis – the price of convenience!

Patients with osteoporosis who are confined to several weeks' bed rest after a fracture frequently sustain more fractures during the subsequent period of mobilisation. A prolonged period of postoperative bed rest should therefore be avoided by implementation of new surgical techniques and the bones should be protected by administration of the appropriate drugs readily available today (e.g., aminobisphosphonates). In addition, there is a close relationship between muscle and bone mass. Moreover, with advancing age, many diseases could be avoided or at least positively influenced by regular exercise and physical activity. It is regrettable that the conveniences of civilisation are won at cost of our bones and that we play a dangerous game in ignoring the increasing trends towards physical inactivity in our children.

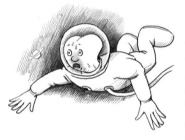

Microgravity. Healthy astronauts must perform special exercises when they are in outer space because of the lack of gravity. Nevertheless, they lose about 1 % of their bone mass every month. Under space flight conditions astronauts experience a loss in bone density at a rate up to ten times faster than that of earth-bound patients with osteoporosis. The decrease in bone during space flight has been extensively studied and used as a model for the decrease in BMD in osteoporosis on earth: in immobilisation due to fractures or paralysis, in the postmenopausal period, and in involutional osteoporosis. Two mechanisms were observed in space flight under microgravity: demineralisation and inhibition of osteoblasts also characterise bone loss here on earth.

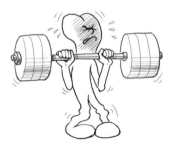

Excessive sport. Female athletes in particular are susceptible to osteoporosis later in life. Constant and lengthy training as well as strict control of diet and weight lead to an extreme reduction in body fat and a drop in levels of oestrogen so that menstrual periods become irregular or cease altogether; consequently, the risk of fractures is clearly increased.

Low body weight. "Slim women, thin bones" – all large studies of risk factors for osteoporosis have confirmed this saying. Underweight women have a high risk of fractures, while overweight women are rarely affected by osteoporosis. This is because the increased weight strengthens the bones while the oestrogen metabolites produced by the fat cells further protect the bones from osteoporosis. After menopause, the hormones produced by the adrenal cortex – androstendione, for example – are metabolised by the fat cells and converted to bone-protecting oestrogen by aromatisation. On the negative side however, overweight has deleterious consequences such as deformities of the vertebrae and "wear and tear" of the joints, especially the knees and ankles. Low body weight with its decrease in bone density and increase in fracture risk affects both men and women equally. For decades our society has broadcast the message that to be thin is attractive, beautiful, and desirable. Embroiled in this "thinness mania," millions of women persist in following misguided attempts at attaining and maintaining thinness at the cost of their bones. It is impossible to consume the nutrients required for bone growth and bone maintenance on a low calorie diet alone. Patients with anorexia nervosa are particularly prone to the development of osteoporosis. In some countries 1%–3% of women are subject to eating disorders, the consequences of which include osteoporosis.

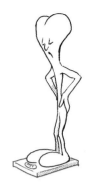

On a diet?
Compensate by supplements, strengthen muscles and bones by regular exercise!

Low lifelong calcium intake. The average adult takes in about 500 mg calcium per day. If there is a decreased calcium intake over years, increased parathyroid hormone levels stimulate bone to release calcium from its stores, and this causes osteoporosis. The greater the calcium intake in childhood and adolescent years, the higher the peak bone mass and bone mass at the menopause, and this makes the bone less susceptible to fracture with normal aging in women as well as in men.

Calcium supply is a lifelong problem. Calcium is not only a substrate for bone formation, it also inhibits bone resorption through its suppressive effect on the blood parathyroid hormone level.

State of depression. Depression by itself is most probably not a cause of osteoporosis, but the accompanying circumstances are. Studies have shown that women with severe longstanding depression have 6% less bone mass than matched controls without depression. Contributory factors are:

► High levels of stress hormones
► Various drugs
► Lack of appetite with inadequate nutrition, and especially
► Reduced physical activity

Women with severe osteoporosis are more prone toward depression and loss of self-esteem. A pronounced or even a beginning dowager's hump can make patients cringe when they look in the mirror.

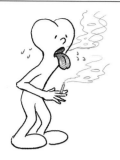

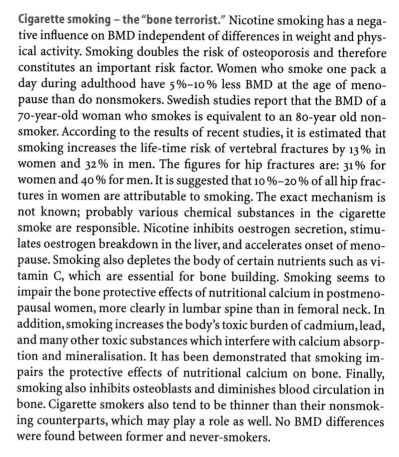

All individuals at risk for osteoporosis or with osteoporosis should stop smoking immediately! If you want to – you can! Smokers have twice as high a risk of hip fractures as non-smokers.

Cigarette smoking – the "bone terrorist." Nicotine smoking has a negative influence on BMD independent of differences in weight and physical activity. Smoking doubles the risk of osteoporosis and therefore constitutes an important risk factor. Women who smoke one pack a day during adulthood have 5%–10% less BMD at the age of menopause than do nonsmokers. Swedish studies report that the BMD of a 70-year-old woman who smokes is equivalent to an 80-year old nonsmoker. According to the results of recent studies, it is estimated that smoking increases the life-time risk of vertebral fractures by 13% in women and 32% in men. The figures for hip fractures are: 31% for women and 40% for men. It is suggested that 10%–20% of all hip fractures in women are attributable to smoking. The exact mechanism is not known; probably various chemical substances in the cigarette smoke are responsible. Nicotine inhibits oestrogen secretion, stimulates oestrogen breakdown in the liver, and accelerates onset of menopause. Smoking also depletes the body of certain nutrients such as vitamin C, which are essential for bone building. Smoking seems to impair the bone protective effects of nutritional calcium in postmenopausal women, more clearly in lumbar spine than in femoral neck. In addition, smoking increases the body's toxic burden of cadmium, lead, and many other toxic substances which interfere with calcium absorption and mineralisation. It has been demonstrated that smoking impairs the protective effects of nutritional calcium on bone. Finally, smoking also inhibits osteoblasts and diminishes blood circulation in bone. Cigarette smokers also tend to be thinner than their nonsmoking counterparts, which may play a role as well. No BMD differences were found between former and never-smokers.

Excessive alcohol intake. Many physicians believe that alcohol intake is bad for bone. However, studies have shown that modest intake is associated with increased oestradiol concentration and therefore with higher bone density and a lower risk of fractures. Therefore, there is no reason to advise individuals who drink alcohol in moderate amounts to stop for reasons of preventing osteoporosis. Alcoholism, however, increases the risk of osteoporosis substantially. Decisive factors are, however, the accompanying poor nutrition, lower weight, hepatic damage, and lower calcium absorption and oestrogen levels. Chronic alcoholism may be 5–10 times more frequent among patients with fractures than among those without fractures. The negative effects of excessive alcohol on bone are seen in women as well as in men.

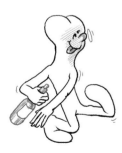

Excessive lipid intake. Hyperlipidemia and an increased susceptibility to lipid oxidation may also constitute risk factors for osteoporosis. In addition, dietary lipids have now been implicated in calcium exclusion, fatty acid metabolism, and osteoblast function.

Nutritional deficiency. Nutrition is an essential factor in the maintenance of bone health, and the following factors are known to be important:

Healthy bones require healthy eating habits. Check labels on food and drink: choose tasty ones with nutritious value!

▶ Minerals: calcium, phosphorus, magnesium, zinc, manganese, copper, boron, silica
▶ Vitamins: D, C, K, B_6, B_{12}, folic acid
▶ Proteins
▶ Essential fatty acids

We frequently underconsume most of these key bone building nutrients, and in a recent survey not a single person consumed 100 % of the Recommended Daily Allowance (RDA) for these nutrients. Especially when insufficient calcium is absorbed from food, it is mobilised from the bones by parathyroid hormones, causing a negative bone balance (i. e., more resorption than formation). In childhood, youth, and pregnancy, it is particularly important to meet the needs of growing bones by appropriate nutrition.

Hormones. An early menopause (natural or surgical) is an important risk factor. Insufficient *testosterone* in men also leads to osteoporosis. Alcoholism and anorexia nervosa can both contribute to testosterone deficiency. Therefore, testosterone levels in the serum should always be investigated in young men with osteoporosis of unknown etiology to detect hypogonadism or testosterone deficiency. Oral *contraceptives* contain a combination of oestrogen and progesterone, and both may increase bone mass. Indeed, there is some evidence that women who have used birth control pills for a long time have stronger bones than those who have not. Oral contraceptives may especially protect some women athletes against the risk of stress fractures.

Medications. Many drugs weaken the bones, and the most important are *cortisone* and its derivates, the glucocorticoids. They are used systemically in many diseases: bronchial asthma, allergies, rheumatic, hematologic, intestinal and immunologic diseases, and transplantation.

If you are taking any drugs, talk to your doctor to see whether they can affect bone loss.

Many diseases and their
therapy effect bones –
consider both!

Patients who are treated with cortisone (or its derivates) for more than
a year develop osteoporosis with a high risk of fractures. There is another long list of medications which weaken the bones on long term
use. These include: lithium, isoniazide, carbamazepin and other antiepileptic drugs, heparin, warfarin and other anticoagulants, antiacids
containing aluminium, and in particular immunosuppressive drugs
such as cyclosporin A. However, thyroid hormones, when given in daily doses of 75–125 µg, probably do not harm the bones. Warfarin com-
petitively inhibits vitamin K, but concern about osteoporosis should
not deter use of anticoagulants for prevention of thromboembolic disorders.

Hospitalisations
are associated with an
increased risk
of falling.

Imbalance, tendency to fall, and obstacles. Almost a third of elderly
people fall at least once a year, but only 10 % will break a bone. Obviously, in addition to the degree of severity of osteoporosis, the type of
fall also determines whether or not a fracture occurs. Protective reflexes – such as stretching out the arms to break a fall – are reduced in older people who also have less energy-absorbing soft tissue around the
hip joints, resulting in an increase in hip fractures in older people. A
very simple test can be used to evaluate a patient's coordination and
thereby the risk of falling and of fractures: the *"rise and walk"* test. The
patient gets up from a chair, walks to a wall 3 meters away, touches it,
and returns to sit on the chair again. If this takes longer than 10 sec-
onds, then there is an increased risk of fracture. Protection against
blows to the side of the hip is afforded by pads which are sewn into the
underwear or worn underneath it. These disperse the impact of the fall
and thus protect the hip joint.

Individuals with higher
muscle mass have less
osteoporosis.

When osteoporosis is already established, various factors – either
health-related or in the environment – may increase the fracture risk.
These include muscular weakness, poor coordination, awkward movements and inadequate protective reactions on falling, excitement,
dizziness, brief fainting attacks, loss of consciousness, Parkinson's disease, reduced vision and alcoholism, and fatigue including drug-induced fatigue (anitdepressive or antihypertensive medication as well
as a variety of sleeping tablets). All of these factors entail a high risk of
falling, as well as decreasing the body's protective mechanisms on falling. Other culprits are obstacles in the home such as telephone and
other wires, stairs, carpets, slippery bathroom mats, lack of grab-bars,
and finally poor lighting.

Early and correct diagnosis is essential for effective therapy. Reliable information concerning the state of bones is absolutely crucial especially if risk factors are already present. The following key questions must be accurately answered:

▶ What is the present bone mass?
▶ What is the present rate of bone loss?
▶ Has physical damage already occurred (fractures, arthroses)?
▶ Are the changes reversible?

Symptoms

Back pain is one of the most frequent reasons for seeking medical advice, and every case of acute or chronic back pain must be thoroughly investigated. Since osteoporosis may be dormant and symptomless for extended periods, the onset of pain may indicate collapse or fracture of a vertebra. On the other hand, osteomalacia is characterised by widespread, early, systemic, and severe bone pain – an important factor in differential diagnosis, which includes numerous other disorders:

▶ Vertebral diseases: inflammatory, degenerative, myelogenous, and neoplastic
▶ Extravertebral diseases: visceral, neurological, muscular, psychosomatic, and neoplastic (e.g., carcinoma of the pancreas).

A detailed *evaluation of back pain* comprises localisation, onset, duration, extent, type, intensity, responsiveness, and sensory/motoric disturbances. Possible underlying causes include:

In suspected osteoporosis: leading questions – correct answers – effective therapy!

Table 6.1. Medical history and physical examination in osteoporosis

Skeletal history	Fractures, pain, deformity, reduced mobility, height loss
Risk factor assessment	
Family history	Osteoporosis, fractures, renal stones
	Age, ethnicity, weight
Medical history	
Reproductive	Menarche > age 15 years, oligo/amenorrhoe, menopause
Diseases	Renal, GI, endocrine, rheumatic, neurologic, eating, depression
Surgery	Gastrectomy, organ transplant, intestinal resection or bypass
Drugs	Glucocorticoids, anticonvulsants, cytotoxic agents, heparin, warfarin, GnRH agonists, lithium
Lifestyle and exercise	Smoking, poor nutrition and exercise, alcohol
Diet and supplements	Frequent dieting, calcium, vitamin D, caffeine, protein
Current medications	Hormones, sedatives, hypertensives, diuretics, nonprescription drugs
Physical examination	
Weight loss, diarrhea	Malabsorption, thyrotoxicosis
Weight gain, hirsutism	Cushing's syndrome
Muscle weakness	Osteomalacia, Cushing's syndrome
Bone pain	Osteomalacia, fracture, malignancy, hyperparathyroidism
Tooth loss	Hypophosphatasia
Joint and lens dislocation	Collagen disorders
Skin pigmentation, stria	Mastocytosis, Cushing's syndrome
Nephrolithiasis	Hypercalcuria, primary hyperparathyroidism

Personal medical history and BMD testing are decisive to determine the best course of osteoporosis prevention and treatment.

▶ Muscular contractions and tension
▶ Vertebral collapse
▶ Protrusion of disc
▶ Ankylosing spondylitis
▶ Bone metastases
▶ Pancreatic tumours
▶ Myocardial infarction

Clinical history and a careful physical examination must include the following:

▶ Loss of height
▶ Posture and bearing
▶ Pain on percussion of spinal processes

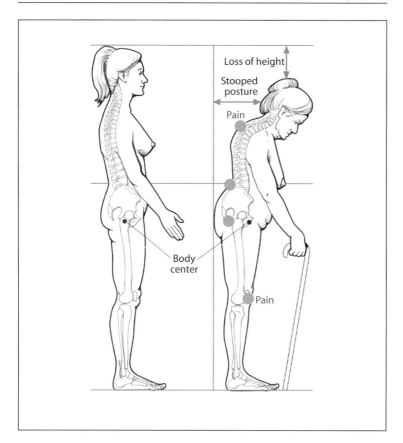

Fig. 6.1. Changes in stature and posture in generalised osteoporosis

▶ Mobility of the vertebral column
▶ Presence of thoracic kyphosis or lumbar scoliosis
▶ Muscle tone and contractions
▶ Signs of congenital osteoporosis (e.g., blue sclerae)

Osteoporosis becomes clinically significant only when the bone fractures!

Acute back pain in osteoporosis is caused by sudden collapse or fracture of a vertebra. Patients often report having heard a snapping or cracking sound in the back. In contrast, chronic pain in osteoporosis is due to inability of the axial skeleton to match up to the demand made on it by muscles, joints, and extremities. The following questions should be answered to make the most comprehensive diagnosis of the pain syndrome: location, nature, timing, and radiation and severity of

Reasons why a patient shrink other than osteoporosis are poor posture, muscle weakness and vertebral disk damage.

the pain, as well as factors that make the pain worse. Neurological features such a persistent nerve root pain or spinal cord syndromes are rare. The massive spinal shrinkage in osteoporosis (>4 cm) is mostly a consequence of the collapse of the thoracic vertebra, but the distance from foot to hip remains constant. Other reasons for moderate decrease in height are poor posture, disk deterioration, and muscle weakness. *Loss of height* can be approximated from the difference between the standing height and the arm span: loss of height occurs only in the spine, with hip-to-heel length remaining constant. When the height of the lumbar spine is reduced, the ribs may come to rest painfully on the bones of the pelvic girdle. A distinctly longer arm span indicates the degree of vertebral bone damage. Loss of height also entails characteristic folds in the skin of the back (*"christmas tree phenomenon"*) as well as a forward-bulge of the abdomen (*"osteoporosis tummy"*). Moreover, the decrease in height of the vertebral bodies results in painful contact between the spinal processes (*"Baastrup-syndrome"* or "kissing spine"). The body's center of gravity is displaced forwards, movement during walking becomes slow and unsure, with small steps to avoid transmitting shocks to the vertebral column. The resulting faulty weight-bearing in turn gives rise to arthroses of the knee-joints (*gonarthrosis*). Moreover, the unsure gait carries with it an increased risk for falls and fractures. The collapse of the thoracic vertebra produces the typical "round" back (*"dowager's hump"*). A good way to measure the degree of "hump" is to measure the distance between the back of the head and the wall when the patient is standing straight up against it. When thoracic kyphosis is marked, it may reduce the thoracic capacity, impairing total lung volume and exercise tolerance, and the patient's chin may come to rest on the sternum.

Shrinking vertebrae start a chain of physical manifestations that may become irreversible – therefore shrinkage must be prevented.

Osteoporosis and Teeth, Skin, and Hair

Teeth are supported by bone: prevent its erosion and preserve your smile!

Metabolic osteopathies involve the whole skeleton, and that includes the teeth and their supporting alveolar bone. Consequently, patients with osteoporosis frequently experience problems with teeth which loosen and fall out due to widening of the canals in which they are situated (alveoli) and loosening of the collagen which holds them in place. Alveolar bone loss also occurs due to periodontitis. Studies have shown that alveolar bone loss and collagen breakdown may be inhibited by administration of aminobisphosphonates. However, attention must of course be paid to the state of the gums.

There is also a connection between "thin, transparent" skin and osteoporosis. Thin skin can be a sign of corticosteroid drug excess or of the Cushing syndrome. Thin skin can best be recognised on the back of the hand, especially when the veins can be seen through it. However, reliable conclusions about bone density cannot be drawn from ultrasound measurements of the thickness of the skin. Fair-haired individuals are more prone to osteoporosis than their darker-skinned and darker-haired counterparts.

Beautiful blondes – beware!

Role of Conventional X-Rays

Skeletal X-rays indicate bone loss only when the density has been reduced by 30 %–40 %; therefore, X-rays are not appropriate for early diagnosis. But they are very useful to reveal previous fractures or compressions. The vertebral bodies exhibit various changes in shape which occur when the cancellous bone is resorbed while the cortex remains intact. Loss of trabecular bone occurs in a predictable pattern. The nonweight-bearing trabeculae are resorbed first and therefore the vertebral bodies typically show a rarefication of the horizontal trabeculae accompanied by a relative accentuation of the vertical trabeculae ("*verticalisation*"), and the presence of reinforcement lines. Furthermore, the cortical rim of the vertebral bodies are accentuated and the bodies may demonstrate a "*picture frame*" or "*empty box*" appearance. Another useful criterion is the *ballooning* of the intervertebral spaces, an indication of the incipient compression of the roof and ground plates (biconcavity of the vertebrae). Schmorl's nodes, which are caused by protrusions of the intervertebral disk into the vertebral body, are common in osteoporosis, although not pathognomonic. The *criteria* used to suggest the presence of osteoporosis on lateral X-rays of the spine include:

Spine radiographs not for early detection but to provide conclusive evidence of manifest osteoporosis, e.g., shape of vertebra.

► Increased radiolucency
► Prominence of vertical trabeculae
► Presence of reinforcement lines
► Thinning of the vertebral endplates
► Presence of compression fractures

Roentgenograms of the thoraco-lumbar region in lateral projection serve two other useful clinical purposes:

▶ Identification of disk degeneration and osteoarthritis, which often cause back pain and thus indicate a different treatment.
▶ Clarification as to why some patients with known severe osteoporosis may have relatively "normal" bone mineral density. Callous formation, degenerative disks, osteoarthritis and calcification of the overlying abdominal aorta may artificially increase bone density measurement.

Spinal X-rays: method of choice for clarification of equivocal results of BMD measurements and for demonstration of numerous conditions responsible for secondary osteoporosis.

It should be emphasised that conventional X-rays of the vertebral column are indispensable in the *investigation of secondary osteoporoses*. Characteristic findings are observed in the following conditions:

▶ *Degenerative-inflammatory conditions of the joints*: Subchondral scleroses with osteophytes or even more extensive ossifications are typical for spondylarthroses and spondylitides.
▶ *Osteomalacia*: "Stout" trabeculae and "Looser's zones" at painful weight-bearing parts of the extremities are characteristic. However, these must be differentiated from osteoporotic fatigue fractures. A bone biopsy in these circumstances provides an unequivocal demonstration of osteomalacia.
▶ *Malignant bone lesions*: Even a slight possibility that a bone lesion is due to a malignant process requires immediate clarification by imaging techniques. MRI is the method of choice in many cases – for example, in multiple myeloma, or suspected metastases in mammary cancer.
▶ *Hyperparathyroidism* (*HPT*): Primary and secondary HPT show similar features on radiology, with the addition of a disturbance of mineralisation in many cases of renal osteodystrophy. In advanced stages there are also pseudocystic clarifications, but the cancellous bone is thicker than in osteoporosis. The vertebra shows a "rugger-jersey-spine" caused by attenuation of the central areas and thickening of the end plates of the vertebral bodies.
▶ *Fluorosis*: The vertebral bodies become completely sclerotic (like marble) with osteophytes and ossification of the vertical bands in the later stages of fluorosis (rarely seen today, as other therapies are now given).

In general, lateral radiographs of the thoracic and lumbar spine should be taken in any patient in whom a vertebral fracture is suspected clinically. Clinical suspicion is heightened by new or worsening back pain, height loss of more than 4 cm, and prominent thoracic kyphosis. A vertebral fracture causes approximately 1 cm loss of height. However, after about age 50, women and men tend to lose height slowly as a result of thinner intervertebral discs and loss of muscle tone in the back. The chance of detecting a vertebral fracture increases with the degree of height loss.

Lateral radiographs provide fast indication of suspected vertebral fractures.

Other Useful Imaging Techniques

Morphometry (Morphometric X-ray absorptiometry, MXA) of the vertebral bodies. X-rays of the thoracic and lumbar spine are taken and the size and contours of the vertebral bodies are measured by means of an automated computer programme. All similar techniques in use today measure the following parameters: the height of the anterior (Ha), medial (Hm), and posterior (Hp) sides of the vertebral body. A 15% or 4 mm reduction in height signifies compression of the vertebral body. Two examples are:

Some DXA devices obtain a lateral image of the entire spine for identifying vertebral fractures based on morphometry. This technique has promise for use in screening for vertebral fractures.

▶ *"Vertebral Deformation Score"* (VDS) according to Kleerekoper: This programme also provides the fracture angle, the projected surface area of the vertebral bodies, and the intervertebral space. Six points are utilised to calculate the deformities of the vertebral bodies. A simple definition of a fracture is the 25% definition: a difference in height of 25% from one measurement to the next. The VDS score is calculated according to the extent of the compression, i. e., VDS 0–3, where VDS 3, for example, signifies a compression fracture effecting Ha, Hm, and Hp.
▶ *"Spine Deformity Index"* according to Minne: It correlates the shape of the vertebral bodies with that of the 4th thoracic vertebra of the same vertebral column.

"Singh-Index." The degree of rarefaction of the tensile groups in the proximal femur corresponds to the fracture risk in this area. Five anatomical groups of trabeculae can be defined which form the basis of the Singh Score. It consists of 3 normal stages and 3–4 stages of increasingly severe osteoporosis (grades 1–7).

The proximal femur and especially the femoral neck require special consideration and have their own indices and parameters to be calculated.

Other parameters of the proximal femur. The *length of the femoral neck* (hip axial length) correlates with the fracture risk at this site independently of the cancellous and compact bone of the proximal femur. The following radiological parameters are useful to calculate the fracture risk in the proximal femur:

▶ Thickness of the medial femoral shaft 3 cm below the trochanter minor
▶ Thickness of the medial cortex at the center of the femoral neck
▶ Femoral head width
▶ Intertrochanteric region width
▶ Acetabular bone width

Microradioscopy. To detect relatively early radiographic signs of osteoporosis, methods such as magnification radiography and radiogrammetry have been developed in the appendicular skeleton. Magnification radiography is a technique to obtain fine detail radiographs of the hands. Radiogrammetry of the metacarpals is a reproducible method of determining the cortical thickness of a bone. This method is inexpensive and readily carried, out but does not detect early osteoporosis.

Focal bone lesions or increased uptake on bone scan require identification!

Bone scan. ^{99m}Tc labelled bisphosphonate is used to detect focal bone lesions and fractures. The whole skeleton can be scanned quickly by this method. Foci of increased uptake in the spine indicate fractures and/or degenerative, inflammatory, or neoplastic lesions. Two days after a fracture, an increased uptake at the site can be expected. However, because of the limited structural details, additional imaging techniques are required for further identification.

High-resolution CT plus image enhancement provide picture of trabecular bone architecture.

Computed Tomography (CT). It is particularly good for analysis of bones, and therefore it was also soon applied for demonstration of the cancellous bone. This can only be done with modern high resolution instruments (sections 0.5 mm thick) together with special picture enhancing facilities, but at the cost of higher exposure to radiation. The value of CT lies in the quantitative computed tomography (QCT), which will be dealt with later.

Magnetic Resonance Imaging (MRI). This method involves no exposure to radiation and is especially adapted for demonstration of the bone marrow. It offers the possibility of identifying both haematopoietic and fatty bone marrow, as well as inflammatory and neoplastic infiltrates. It is the method of choice for demonstration of myeloma, lymphoma, and metastases, as well as localised edematous processes (transient osteoporosis and early stages of Sudeck's disease). It is the ideal method to distinguish between an osteoporotic fracture and one due to spinal metastases. In addition, the diagnostic capability is greatly enhanced by application of special gradient echo sequences and by the use of contrast media.

MRI: the best method for investigation of all conditions affecting the bone marrow and subsequently the bone.

CHAPTER 7

Bone Mineral Density (BMD): The Crucial Diagnostic Parameter

Why Measure Bone Mineral Density?

Bone density is the most objective, reliable and quantifiable parameter for diagnosis of osteoporosis and to monitor therapy. It is crucial for early detection and prevention due to its accurate prediction of fracture risk.

The early diagnosis of osteoporosis, before occurrence of fractures, can only be made by means of bone density measurements (bone mineral density tests, BMD). These measure bone density at various skeletal sites and thereby enable a prediction of risk of later fracture. A 10 % decrease in bone density doubles the fracture risk for the vertebral body and trebles it for the hip joint. If a fracture has already occurred, this test is used to confirm the diagnosis of osteoporosis and determine its degree of severity. BMD provides the following information:

▶ Detects osteopenia and/or osteoporosis before occurrence of a fracture
▶ Predicts risk for later development of osteoporosis
▶ Indicates the rate of bone loss – progression – in sequential measurements
▶ Documents the efficacy or failure of therapy
▶ Increases compliance of both doctor and patient

The relation between BMD and fracture risk is well established. The association between bone density (measured at hip and lumbar spine) and hip fracture is three times stronger than that between cholesterol levels and heart disease. Currently, a bone density measurement remains the best and most readily quantifiable method for assessing fracture risk and skeletal response to different treatments.

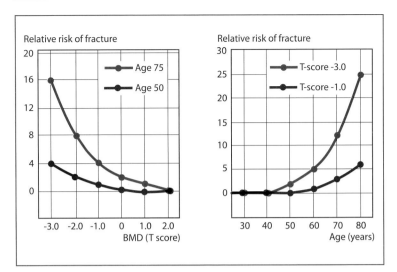

Fig. 7.1. Relative risk of fracture according to BMD and age

Table 7.1. Techniques for measuring bone mineral density (BMD)

Method	Precision (%)	Accuracy (%)	Scan time (min)	Radiation dose (mrems)

Dual-energy X-ray Absorptiometry (DXA)
  Lumbar spine AP
  Lumbar spine lateral
  Proximal radius
  Distal radius
  Proximal femur
  Total body
	1–2	3–5	2–8	1–3

Quantitative Computed Tomography (QCT)
  Lumbar spine
  Radius
	2–10	5–20	10–15	100–1,000

Quantitative Ultrasound (QUS)
  Calcaneus
  Phalanges
  Patella
	–	2–8	5–10	0

Which Instruments to Use?

If there is a choice: choose DXA, the most widely used and popular instrument! DXA is the gold standard of BMD measurement technology.

The *bone mineral content (BMC)* is measured in grams, and the *bone mineral density (BMD)* in g/cm^2 (area) or g/cm^3 (volumetric). The precision and accuracy of a measurement depend on:

▶ Type of instrument (pencil or fan beam techniques)
▶ Regular (daily) check and setting of the instrument
▶ Cooperation of the patient (must keep still)
▶ Exact adjustment of the instrument by the investigator
▶ Degree of osteoporosis: the less the bone mass the more inaccurate the measurement!

Dual Energy X-ray Absorptiometry (DEXA, DXA, rarely also called QDR, DPX, DER). Today DEXA is the most completely developed, reliable, and popular method in use, the "gold standard." DEXA was developed in the 1980s and its widespread use began in 1988. The skeletal site is exposed to two X-ray beams of different intensity, and the mineral con-

Fig. 7.2. DXA unit for measurement of bone density in the lumbar spine and the hips. Note posture of patient required for accurate measurement

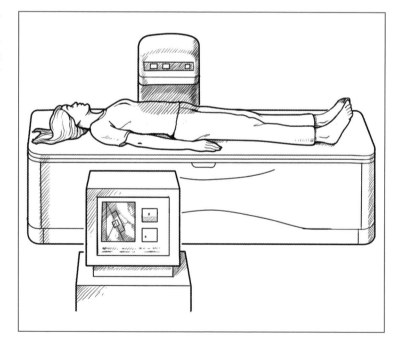

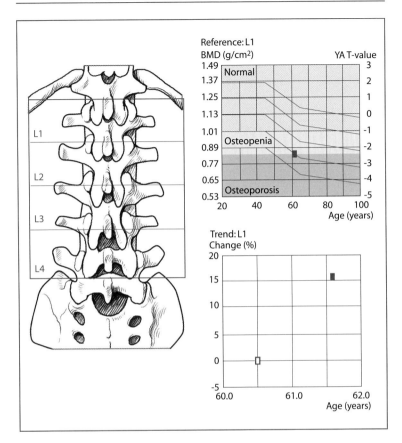

Reference: L1
BMD (g/cm²)

Trend: L1
Change (%)

Fig. 7.3. DEXA of the lumbar spine (L1-L4). *Upper right*: Note T-score of −2.5, a borderline value between osteopenia and osteoporosis. *Lower right*: Positive effect of alendronate on bone density with 15% increase after 1 year of therapy

tent of the bone is calculated by means of computer programs from the amount of radiation. Using the results of the two measurements, the effects of the soft tissue components (different quantities of muscle and fatty tissue) can be calculated and discarded. DXA can measure central (hip and spine) and peripheral (forearm) sites, and can even perform a total body scan ("full body DXA scanner").

The hip joint and the lumbar spine are routinely measured from the front (AP) or the side (lateral). The combined evaluation of these two measurements improves the assessment of a patient's bone mineral status and the fracture prediction, especially in cases with anatomic variations, severe degenerative changes, or fractures. The measurements of the lumbar spine are not confined to the vertebral bodies,

Accurate results depend on careful measurement!

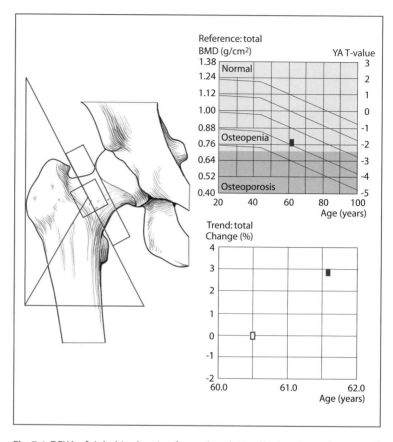

Fig. 7.4. DEXA of right hip showing femoral neck, Ward's triangle, trochanter, and shaft. *Upper right*: Note T-score of −2.0, within osteopenic range. *Lower right*: Positive effect of raloxifene on bone density with 3 % increase after 1 year of therapy

Both total hip and lumbar vertebrae are measured for greater accuracy. The diagnosis is based on the lowest T-score.

they also include the arches and spinous processes, which have a considerable quantity of compact bone. The International Society of Clinical Densitometry (ISCD) suggests measurement of at least two sites if possible and recommends that diagnosis is based on the lowest T-score. It suggests using the L2-L4 average measurement rather than a single vertebra if possible. In measurements of the hip, either the total hip or the femoral neck measurement is used, whichever is the lowest standard deviation. To summarise, the important advantages of DXA are:

► It is not invasive, the patient remains clothed and it is therefore not a burden to the patient.
► It is very quickly carried out (5–10 min).
► It is cost-effective.
► It has a very low radiation dose (1–3 mRem equivalent to 1/10–1/100 of a normal X-ray film).
► It measures those skeletal areas most vulnerable to osteoporosis and to fractures – the lumbar spine and the hips.
► The measurements are accurate and therefore ideal for follow-up and control investigations (accuracy error 1%–10%, precision 1%)
► It is recognised by the WHO as the standard method for definition of diagnosis.

The results of the measurement of the lumbar vertebral bodies 1–4 are expressed separately as well as in combination, by which single, possibly defective vertebrae can be excluded. Many factors dealing mainly with variations in density in the spine and/or in neighbouring soft tissues can give misleading values and must be considered in the results. In really difficult cases, measurement of the lumbar spine may have to be abandoned and only the bones of the hip joint measured. However, there may also be variations in density in the proximal femur so that great care must be taken to measure the same areas in sequential investigations. The only real disadvantage of DEXA is that everything in the selected area is included. Sometimes it may be difficult to decide what an ossification is due to (for example aorta, calcified lymph nodes or muscles, spondylophytes, etc.). Other X-ray-dense substances such as metal-fasteners on clothes, X-ray-dense contrast media, or calcium tablets may also be included in the overall measurement. These "pitfalls" can be recognised and subsequently avoided by a prior X-ray of the skeletal area to be measured. Recent developments in instrumentation enable lateral measurement, and by means of picture enhancement the vertebral bodies and the hip are clearly displayed. Because of its high precision, it is wise for premenopausal women to get a baseline DEXA scan that can serve as a reference value to determine loss of bone density after menopause.

Two terms, T-score and Z-score, are commonly used to report DXA results and both of these rely on a *standard deviation* (*SD*) for the measurement. SD represents the normal variability in a measurement in a population: the difference between the 5th and the 95th percentile of a group covers about 4 SDs. One SD of the hip or spine BMD corresponds to about 10%–15% of the mean value.

If you want to know exactly how strong the bones really are, make a bone density test by DXA.

▶ *Z-score* is the number of SDs below (minus) or above (plus) the mean BMD value for people of the same age ("age- and sex-matched" controls).

▶ *T-score* is the number of SDs below or above the mean value of BMD for young (20–30-year old) adults ("peak bone density").

Because BMD declines with age at all sites, after age 30 the T-scores are lower than the Z-scores, and the differences increase with age. By definition, diagnosis of osteoporosis is based on a T-score of <–2,5 SD.

Single energy X-ray absorptiometry (SXA). This method is still used today to measure the bones of the ankle because of the paucity of surrounding soft tissue.

QCT provides separate measurements of cortical and trabecular bone and may be especially valuable in older people (men!).

Quantitative computed tomography (QCT). This is an established technique to measure BMD of the lumbar spine and appendicular skeleton. Moreover, it provides cross-sectional images and therefore separate measurements of trabecular and cortical bone as well as true volumetric mineral density in g/cm^3. In clinical studies, QCT has been used for assessment of vertebral fracture risk. The method is usually applied to the spine to measure trabecular bone in consecutive vertebrae (Th 12-L4). The measurement takes about 20 min and has a relatively high radiation exposure of about 100–1,000 mSv. The region of interest (ROI) is either manually or automatically positioned. QCT can be performed in single-energy (SEQCT) or dual-energy (DEQCT) modes, which differ in precision, accuracy, and radiation exposure. The presence of marrow fat in the vertebral bodies may cause an underestimation of BMD by 10%-15%. The values obtained by direct measurement and by means of a "calibration phantom" should not be reported as T-score but they are calculated as hydroxyapatite mass per volume:

Normal	>120 HA/cm^3
Osteopenia	120–80 HA/cm^3
Osteoporosis	<80 HA/cm^3

Small instruments are available for small bones (fingers), but they are site-specific only.

Special, small instruments are used to measure bone density in the fingers and the wrist (*pQCT*). The values obtained, however, cannot be considered as representative to the skeleton as a whole, even though they do give accurate values for the bones measured. For example, cancellous bone in the radius may show osteoporosis in density measurements but may be nowhere near that of the lumbar vertebrae or the hips. The future of computed tomography lies in the field of direct visualisation of trabecular bone architecture by high-resolution and 3 dimensional (volumetric) imaging – *3D-CT.* However, this development does entail a greater amount of radiation.

On the horizon:
3D-CT for direct visualisation of the trabecular network!

Radiographic absorptiometry (RA). This technique determines BMD through computed analysis of hand radiographs. RA has proven to be a practical, inexpensive, and rapid way do evaluate BMD:

RA is especially useful in paediatrics to determine skeletal age and development.

▶ Two postero-anterior radiographs are taken of the hand, one at 50 kVp and the other at 60 kVp using nonscreen film.
▶ The films are sent to a central laboratory where they are digitised by a high-resolution imaging system.
▶ BMD is calculated in arbitrary units using the aluminium reference wedge as a calibration material.
▶ RA measures both trabecular and cortical bone.
▶ RA has a high precision and accuracy.
▶ The radiation exposure of about 100 mrems is lower than that of QCT but higher than that of DEXA.
▶ RA has a high sensitivity in predicting low bone mass of the lumbar spine and femoral neck (90 % and 82 %, respectively)
▶ RA plays an important role in paediatric osteology as radiographs of the hand are taken routinely in paediatric individuals for the purpose of determining skeletal age and development.

Quantitative Ultrasound (QUS). This is already used successfully in many different conditions. The FDA has approved QUS of bone for its diagnostic value in osteoporosis and related fractures. The behaviour of these ultrasound waves in bone differs greatly from that of X-rays. The absorption, speed, and the reflection in bone and from its surface are all measured. Two major parameters are used in measuring bone by QUS:

QUS now accepted as screening test to estimate fracture risk.

▶ Speed of sound through bone (transit velocity, SOS)
▶ Attenuation of sound as it passes through bone (broad-band ultrasound attenuation, BUA dB/MHz)

Some instruments combine SOS and BUA to formulate a clinical index (quantitative ultrasound index, QUI). The skeletal part to be measured is placed between the ultrasound transmitter and receiver. Consequently, this method is very suitable for easily accessible bones: calcaneus, radius, tibia, and phalanges. It is currently accepted that the QUS results are influenced mainly by three parameters:

▶ Microarchitecture of bone
▶ Mineral constituents of bone matrix
▶ Elastic modulus

Recent studies have shown that QUS of the calcaneus is a predictor of hip fracture risk, independent of femoral BMD, and that this technology can discriminate between normal and osteoporotic subjects. For every SD decrease in BUA of the calcaneus, the risk of hip fracture increases twofold, comparable with the results of DEXA. QUS is becoming increasingly popular because of the absence of exposure to radiation and the simplicity of application. An additional advantage is that the cortical and cancellous bone are described separately. These advantages account for the fact that QUS is now widely applied as a screening test, though it cannot yet replace DEXA measurements of the spine and hips. It must be emphasised that normal values for the fingers using QUS do not rule out the possibility of a severe osteoporosis of the spine or hips. Conversely, if the phalanges show osteoporotic values then this should be regarded as a manifestation of generalised osteoporosis and DEXA of the lumbar spine and/or hips should be carried out for clarification and WHO classification. Measurements of the fingers are especially indicated in patients with rheumatic disorders involving the hands. At present, QUS is not recommended for monitoring of treatment.

Which Bones to Measure?

A fundamental rule states that "the result of a bone density measurement applies only to the particular site measured." Osteoporosis does not effect all the bones of the skeleton to the same degree. Bones with a high proportion of cancellous (trabecular) bone, such as the vertebrae and hip bones, are the first victims and these bones are also the first to suffer fractures. Concordance of bone mass between different skeletal sites in individual patients increases in the elderly population. However, even in the elderly female population, measuring only the hip to make a diagnosis of osteoporosis (<-2.5 SD) will detect slightly less than 50 % of the affected people, whereas measuring multiple skeletal sites in this population will detect nearly 80 % of the affected people. Therefore, the lumbar vertebrae and hip bones are always measured according to a precise, topographical plan. The more sites measured, the higher the likelihood that a diagnosis of osteoporosis will be made. Of course, also the reverse is true: if only one peripheral site is measured, there is a much higher probability of missing osteoporosis. The peripheral techniques are quick and easy to use, but they are not appropriate for initial diagnosis or to measure response to therapy.

Lumbar vertebrae are measured individually and together, but fractured or otherwise deformed vertebrae are excluded.

Five areas are measured in the *hip joint:*

▶ Femoral neck
▶ Trochanter
▶ Intertrochanteric region
▶ Ward's triangle.
▶ Total

Subsequently, when the bone density is checked for monitoring therapy or progression of disease, it is crucial to measure exactly the same areas again.

The *ankle* is also a good site to measure, because of its content of trabecular bone and its accessibility. When done by QUS, differences in rarefaction of the trabecular network along stress lines must be taken into account, and the exact same area must be measured for subsequent monitoring. DEXA does not have this drawback since the whole ankle is measured and the exact area is illustrated.

In the past, the *radius* was frequently measured but the significance of the results is reduced because of the variable amounts of cancellous and cortical bone and of surrounding soft tissues. The same applies to pQCT and QUS of the radius. However, one advantage of pQCT is that the architecture of the distal radius is displayed.

Worried patients frequently come into outpatient clinics and produce the results of density measurements of the fingers together with the diagnosis "severe osteoporosis with very high risk of fractures."

Measuring BMD at the hip and/or lumbar spine is the best way of predicting fractures.

Identical sites must be measured to monitor therapy and/or progression of disease.

Never rely only on a peripheral bone measurement for diagnosis of osteoporosis.

Subsequent density measurement of spine and hip may reveal normal values. The opposite may also occur – normal bone density in the fingers with severe osteoporosis in the axial skeleton and multiple fractures of the vertebral bodies. Such situations simply indicate different bone density in different parts of the skeleton! The lesson to be drawn from this is that the diagnosis of generalised osteoporosis must never be based on the result of a peripheral bone density measurement. In addition, DEXA density measurements to monitor therapy must always be made on the same skeletal site, preferably by the same instrument (DEXA) at yearly intervals.

Investigations of the *whole skeleton* to determine bone mineral content are only made in clinical trials.

Indications for BMD

Until recently, the diagnosis of osteoporosis was largely based on history, X-rays, and clinical symptoms, especially fractures. The clinical relevance of quantitative bone density measurements are based upon two important assumptions:

▶ That bone density is related to fracture risk
▶ That treatments to increase bone mass can be given

Two crucial facts determine indications for BMD:
• Its ability accurately to determine fracture risk
• The availability of therapy to increase BMD.

Indeed, with the introduction of quantitative techniques of bone densitometry, the diagnosis of osteoporosis can now already be established in the early asymptomatic phase of the disease. Low bone density is accepted as the most important predictor of fragility fractures, comparable with blood pressure and cholesterol as reliable predictors of subsequent cardiovascular disease. Nevertheless, density measurements are not yet recommended as a screening procedure. However, for health conscious individuals this test is just as important as other generally established investigations. It is cheap, simple to perform, and facilitates subsequent diagnosis and monitoring.

Indications for bone density measurements. Any individual with risk factors should have a bone density measurement, for example a postmenopausal woman who does not take HRT or its equivalent, a woman with early menopause or a family history of osteoporosis, or men with decreased levels of androgens. According to the *National Os-*

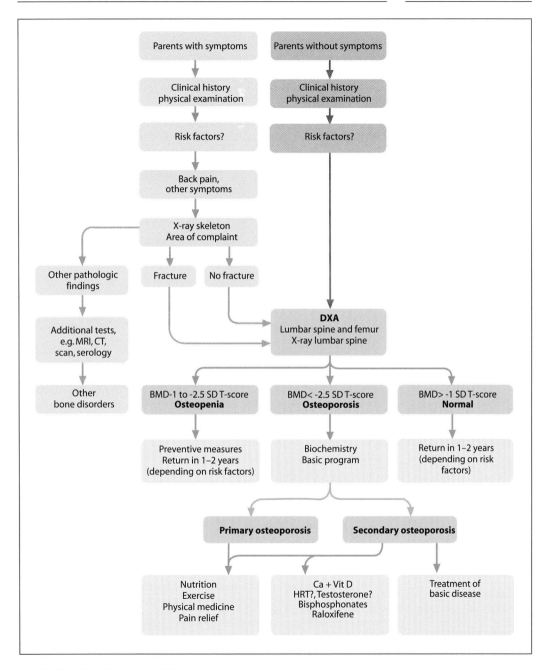

Fig. 7.5. Algorithm for diagnostic investigation and treatment of osteoporosis

teoporosis Foundation (*NOF*) a BMD measurement is recommended for:

▶ All women >65 years regardless of additional risk factors
▶ All women <65 years with one or more risk factors
▶ All postmenopausal women with fractures
▶ All women contemplating osteoporosis therapy and whose decision depends on the result of BMD
▶ All women undergoing protracted hormone therapy
▶ Indications for men are given in Chapter 19
  Additional indications:
▶ Age-related decrease in height
▶ Back pain of obscure origin
▶ Slim smokers
▶ Previous fractures
▶ Diseases of joints which limit movement
▶ Long-term use (>6 months) of drugs such as cortisone, warfarin, heparin, or antiepileptic drugs
▶ Hyperthyroidism and hyperparathyroidism
▶ Posttransplantation, especially of kidney, liver, heart, and lungs
▶ Chronic diseases and operations which can lead to bone loss, e.g., gastric and intestinal resections
▶ Anorexia nervosa
▶ Chronic renal insufficiency

The method of choice to monitor therapy is BMD by DEXA. Since radiation exposure is very low, it can be done annually or even biennially, and there is no need for isolation during testing.

Bone density measurement by DEXA is currently the only reliable method to document the effects of therapy on osteoporosis. Decrease in the incidence of fractures is another. Moreover, annual BMD measurements increase the patient's compliance (though this is now less of a problem). Clinical trials have documented significant increases in bone density under therapy with bisphosphonates after 3 months in the vertebrae and 1 year in the hips. Biannual measurements should be carried out in high-risk patients, for example, those on corticoid therapy or patients with rapid bone loss (as indicated by biochemical parameters).

Bone Densitometry in Children: Now Readily Available

So far, little attention has been paid to the analysis of bone mass during growth. Four current techniques are now employed in paediatrics:

▶ The most widely used: DEXA
▶ The most versatile: QCT
▶ The newest: QUS
▶ Under investigation: MRI

The preferred sites for scanning include the lumbar spine, the hip, and the whole body but also peripheral sites such as the forearm and the hand. The radiation dose is extremely low, about 1 µSv for lumbar spine and 4 µSv for whole skeleton scans. In children, the precision ranges from 1%–2.5% in most studies. Although various manufacturers have developed special software to be used in paediatrics, this software requires longer scanning time, which makes cooperation from children difficult. Correct positioning is also of the utmost importance in scanning children. Recently leading manufacturers have proposed a standardised software for measurements of the lumbar spine. The low costs, availability, and ease of use are the main advantages of DEXA. With respect to QUS, SOS values have been obtained at the calcaneus, patella, and phalanges of the thumb, whereas BUA values in children are mainly obtained at the calcaneus. These measurements seem to be correlated more with bone size than with changes in the amount, density, or geometry of bone.

DEXA is also good for children and bone size does not count, as with other methods.

BMD Measurement: Not a Scary Procedure, Nothing to Be Afraid of!

Low bone mass is the most important objective predictor of fracture risk, and BMD measurement is simple to perform for the patient. Considering that the "natural" exposure to radiation is about 2,400 µSv, for example 100 µSv during a transatlantic flight, then the 10 µSv of a DEXA measurement is so low that it is the most suitable for monitoring. For comparison, the radiation dose of currently used techniques are listed:

Bone density tests (DXA) are extremely low in radiation, so the technician can stay in the room during the scan.

X-ray, lateral lumbar spine	1,000 μSv
QCT	100 μSv
DXA PA pencil beam	10 μSv
DXA PA fan beam	1 μSv
pQCT	1 μSv
QUS	0 μSv

CHAPTER 8 Laboratory Investigations in Osteoporosis: Are They Needed?

Which Tests Are Necessary?

The parameters usually tested in blood and urine are within normal limits in primary osteoporosis. The significance of laboratory tests therefore lies mainly in recognising secondary osteoporoses. Consequently, the following "basic" laboratory screening tests should be carried out regularly:

Routine blood and urine tests are required for screening to identify or rule out secondary osteoporosis at any age.

▶ Erythrocyte sedimentation rate
▶ Complete blood count
▶ Calcium and phosphate (serum)
▶ Alkaline phosphatase (serum)
▶ Glucose (serum/urine)
▶ Transaminases and GT (serum)
▶ Creatinine (serum)

And when the appropriate indications are present:
▶ T_3, T_4, and TSH
▶ Oestrogen and/or testosterone levels
▶ Vitamin D metabolites
▶ Parathormone
▶ Protein electrophoresis and immunoelectrophoresis

It is important to note that 20 % of women and up to 64 % of men with osteoporosis have diseases linked to osteoporosis.

Table 8.1. Laboratory tests for the evaluation of secondary osteoporoses. *S*, serum, *U*, urine

Basic tests	Diseases	Additional tests to include
Complete blood count	Malabsorption	PTH, vitamin D, calcium (S)
		Ferritin, vitamin B12
	Multiple myeloma	Bone marrow biopsy
		Protein electrophoresis (S,U)
	Leukaemia	Blood smear
	Bone metastases	PSA, Ca15–3, CEA
Thyroid-stimulating Hormone (TSH)	Hyperthyroidism	Thyroxine (T4), T3
Glucose (S,U)	Diabetes mellitus	Oral glucose tolerance test
Cortisol (S)	Cushing's syndrome	ACTH, dexamethasone test
	Addison's disease	ACTH
HIV-antibody	AIDS	Infection diagnosis
HLA B-27	Ankylosing spondylitis	CRP
Testosterone in men	Hypogonadism	SHBG, LH, FSH, Prolactin
Calcium (S)	Hyperparathyroidism	PTH
	Malabsorption	Complete blood count
	Morbus Crohn	PTH, vitamin D
	Celiac disease	Alkaline phosphatase, gliadin
	Osteomalacia	PTH, vitamin D
		Alkaline phosphatase
Alkaline phosphatase	Chronic renal failure	PTH, calcium, phosphate (S)
	Osteomalacia	PTH, vitamin D
		Calcium (S)
Protein electrophoresis	Multiple myeloma	Complete blood count
		Bone marrow biopsy
Liver enzymes	Haemochromatosis	Iron, ferritin (S)
	Alcoholic liver disease	
	Primary biliary cirrhosis	Antibodies
Creatinine	Chronic renal failure	PTH, calcium, phosphate (S)
Histamine 24 h U	Mastocytosis	Bone marrow biopsy

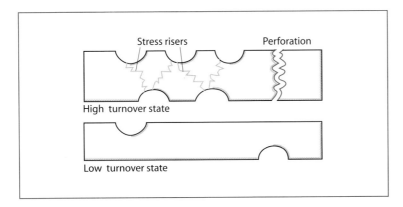

Significance of Markers of Bone Turnover

The measurements of bone turnover in daily practice are essential for the diagnosis and monitoring of progressive bone diseases such as metastases or Paget's disease of bone. However, bone markers cannot be used to diagnose osteoporosis, although they may help to answer some important clinical questions:

Bone turnover markers cannot be used to diagnose osteoporosis.

▶ Predicting the future rate of bone loss (high or low bone turnover)
▶ Predicting the risk of osteoporotic fractures
▶ Monitoring response to therapy

Metabolites of bone remodelling, i.e., resorption and formation by which bone is constantly maintained and renewed, pass into the blood stream and from there into the urine. These products can be identified biochemically as well as their levels in blood and urine which indicate "high turnover" or "low turnover" osteoporoses. Bone turnover markers represent either enzymes involved in bone formation (produced by osteoblasts) and resorption (generated by osteoclasts) or the formation and degradation products of bone matrix metabolism (such as type I collagen). Bone markers do not replace bone density measurements for the diagnosis of osteoporosis. However, these markers may give information about the future risk for bone loss and fragility fractures. Changes in bone formation in response to therapy are relatively slow, starting after some weeks and reaching a plateau after several months, while bone resorption decreases rapidly a few days after start-

Table 8.2. Biochemical markers of bone turnover

Bone resorption	Bone formation
Blood	**Blood**
Tartrate-resistant acid phosphatase(TRAP)	Total or bone-specific alkaline phosphatase
Free pyridinoline or deoxypyridninoline	Osteocalcin
N- or C-telopeptide of type I collagen	Procollagen I C-and N-terminal extension peptides
Cross-links	Osteocalcin
Urine	
Fasting urine calcium-to-creatinine ratio	
Pyridinoline and deoxypyridinoline	
Glycosides of hydroxylysine	
Pyridinoline and desoxypyridinoline	
N- and C-telopeptides of type I collagen	

Markers of bone formation reflect osteoblastic activity.

ing an antiresorptive therapy such as a bisphosphonate and reaches a nadir after a few weeks.

Parameters of bone formation are bone specific alkaline phosphatase (bone ALP), osteocalcin (OC), and osteonectin. These are produced by osteoblasts (possibly also by endothelial cells) and reflect their activity. ALP is also produced in various tissues, including liver and kidney. Bone-specific ALP can be distinguished by immunoassays with high specificity. Osteocalcin shows a diurnal rhythm and only about 50 % is released into the circulation, while the remaining 50 % is incorporated into hydroxyapatite. OC reflects total bone turnover, both resorption and formation. The serum concentrations of the C- and N-terminal propeptides of type I procollagen (PICP and PINC) reflect changes in synthesis of new collagen, both by osteoblasts in bone and by fibroblasts in other connective tissues. PICP and PIN are completely secreted into the circulation.

High levels of bone resorption markers have been associated with increased fracture risk.

Parameters of bone resorption consist primarily of collagen degradation products such as "cross links" which are released into the blood stream and then excreted into the urine. They appear to predict the risk of hip fracture in elderly women independently of bone density. Studies have shown that women with high levels of bone resorption have about a 1.5 to 3-fold increased risk of hip or nonvertebral fractures. Desoxypyridinoline and cross-link telopeptides of type I collagen are the two most frequently investigated. Telopeptides are distinguished by their terminals: amino- (*NTX-OSTEOMARK*) and

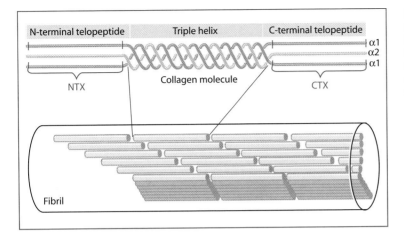

Fig. 8.2. Molecular structure and organisation of collagen into fibrils. Note position of end terminal CTX and NTX, used as biochemical markers of collagen break-down in the serum

carboxy- (*CTX-CROSSLAPS*). Variations in diurnal rhythm and the effect of meals must be taken into account when results of these tests are evaluated. Both NTX and CTX show a significant response to antiresorptive therapy and are currently considered to be the best parameters of bone resorption. Serum NTX concentrations are elevated in chronic renal failure, which must of course be taken into account.

Bone sialoprotein (*BSP*) also appears to be a sensitive marker of bone turnover. Furthermore, BSP is thought to play an important role in attraction and growth of tumour cells in the bone marrow (e.g. breast cancer and multiple myeloma).

Hydroxyproline should no longer be used as a marker of bone metabolism because of its lack of specificity. Its urinary excretion is also influenced by the breakdown of collagen in other sites and by dietary collagen intake.

Excretion of *calcium* in a 24 h urinary specimen is also not an accurate reflection of bone resorption, because it depends on the renal threshold for calcium reabsorption and the dietary calcium intake.

Results of bone markers before starting a treatment are not useful predictors of response to treatment. It is also not clear if patients with high bone turnover are more likely to gain more bone under therapy. Some studies have demonstrated that patients with the largest decreases in markers of bone resorption during treatment with alendronate tend to have the greatest increases in BMD. Nevertheless, changes in markers during treatment must be interpreted with care. The

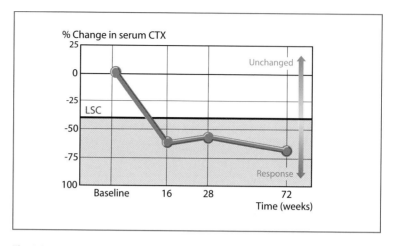

Fig. 8.3. Bone marker response to antiresorptive agents. A decrease below the least significant change (LSC) is regarded as statistically significant

Patients may benefit from therapy without significant decreases in markers or increases in BMD providing the fracture risk is reduced.

results of each patient must be compared with the "*least significant change*" (LSC). The LSC is the minimum change that must be seen in an individual patient to be at least 95% sure that the change is "real" and not caused by biological or laboratory variations. The LSC is about 25% for most formation markers and 40%–65% for most resorption markers. About 65% of patients treated with oestrogen or bisphosphonates have changes in bone resorption markers that are greater than the LSC. In contrast, raloxifene and calcitonin are associated with smaller changes in bone resorption. However, patients may benefit from reductions in risk of fracture even if they do not have reductions in bone markers or improvements in bone density. In these cases with little or no change while taking medication it is important to check carefully:

▶ If the patient is taking the medication at all
▶ If the patient is taking the drug as prescribed
▶ If there are secondary causes of osteoporosis

The advantage of monitoring treatment with markers is that changes in levels can be observed within weeks of starting therapy, at a time when patients are most likely to discontinue medication. It is important to emphasise that the specimens are taken at about the same time of day and with the patient in a fasting state. Furthermore, indices of bone turnover may show seasonal and circadian variations. Unfortunately, studies to determine whether compliance is improved by monitoring the treatment have not yet been published.

When Is a Bone Biopsy Indicated?

Before dealing with this question, it should be clearly stated the diagnosis of osteoporosis is based on clinical findings and bone density measurements. In addition, it should be pointed out that normal bone histology in an iliac crest biopsy does not exclude osteoporosis elsewhere, for example, in the axial skeleton. Nevertheless, a bone biopsy is sometimes required for investigation of other disorders of bone.

Obtaining a bone biopsy nowadays is a relatively simple procedure and nearly always without complications. There are a number of new improved biopsy needles available, as well as up-to-date techniques for processing bone biopsies from fixation and embedding to histology and immunohistology. These methods provide optimal biopsy sections for evaluation of the overall structure of cortex and trabeculae, architecture of the cancellous bone, bone cells and remodelling, mineralisation, and haematopoiesis. In clinical trials these parameters are also evaluated quantitatively by histomorphometry.

Bone biopsies are indicated in the investigation of secondary osteoporoses; in these conditions they provide essential information. When a disturbance of mineralisation is suspected, histological evidence can be obtained by means of bone biopsies. In renal osteodystrophy (ROD) bone biopsies provide essential information required to determine the type of ROD and the severity of the lesions. Though in widespread use, PTH levels in serum are not necessarily predictive of the underlying bone disease which can, however, be readily assessed by bone biopsy. In addition, estimation of the histological aspects of bone and its cells enable correlation with parameters of bone remodelling and with age. Disorders of the bone marrow and/or a malignant metastatic process are additional indications.

To summarise, a bone biopsy is no longer necessary for the demonstration of uncomplicated bone loss in primary osteoporosis; it has been replaced by the noninvasive BMD measurements. When other underlying causes are suspected or established, a bone biopsy may provide essential information.

Always check for secondary causes of osteoporosis, in many of which a bone biopsy may provide essential information, e.g., in renal, haematologic and oncologic disorders.

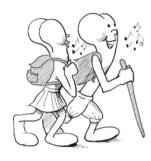

Maintenance of healthy bones and thereby avoidance of osteoporotic fractures can be achieved by institution and adherence to a specific *plan of action*, a programme of nine specific steps for the prevention of bone loss. These *self-help measures* are just as important for people who do not have osteoporosis because they reduce the risk of developing the disease. There is one condition for success of the plan – a sine qua non! – the individual him/herself must have the will power to start immediately and the perseverance to continue! The goal for the twenty-first century:

Population – the quality of life up!
Authorities – the cost of health care down!

Step 1: A Calcium-Rich Diet

The first essential is a calcium-rich diet, which can be achieved by everybody. But some studies reveal that 80 % of American women do not get adequate amounts of calcium.

Calcium is the most important mineral for prevention and treatment of osteoporosis. An adult has over 1 kg of calcium in the body, 99 % of which is in the skeleton. A fifth of total bone mass is calcium.

▶ Prevention of osteoporosis begins in *childhood*. M. Drugay defined osteoporosis as a "paediatric disease with geriatric consequences." As the skeleton develops and grows, a calcium-rich diet provides the building blocks required to reach a peak bone mass at about 25 years. During this period children and young people need about four times as much calcium as adults per kilogram of body weight. Depending on age, 500–1,500 mg of calcium should be ingested daily.

▶ Even weight-conscious *teenagers* can achieve this goal by means of a calcium-rich, fat-poor diet including low-fat milk, cheese and

Table 9.1. Suggested calcium intakes

Age groups	Amount mg/day
Infants	
0–6 months	210
6–12 months	270
Children	
1–3 years	500
4–8 years	800
9–18 years	1,500
Adults	
19–50 years	1,200
51 years and older	1,500
Pregnant and lactating women	1,500

yoghurt, and calcium-rich drinks – fruit juice – and bread. Just one cup of yoghurt gets most girls a third of the way to their daily requirement. We know that the early to mid-teens are a critical time in bone formation. One clinical trial found that by the age of 16 young women have already reached about 95 % of their mothers' premenopausal bone density.

▶ The requirement for calcium is particularly high during *pregnancy* and *lactation*, about 1,200–1,500 mg a day.

▶ It is not too late to start a bone-conscious diet even after *menopause*, especially since there is a dramatic increase in bone loss at this time. Clinical trials have demonstrated that 80 % of postmenopausal women require more than 800 mg calcium ingested daily in food. During this period of increased resorption, the daily intake should be 1,500 mg. Some evidence points to greater effectiveness perimenopausally than postmenopausally in reducing bone loss. In other words, preventive measures should be instituted before cessation of ovarian function.

Osteoporosis is not an inevitable part of the ageing process. It can be prevented!

Sufficient calcium can be obtained by means of a *"bone-friendly" diet*:

▶ *Milk and milk products* are rich in calcium, especially low-fat milk and hard cheeses. The harder the cheese, the more calcium it contains. Soft cheeses also frequently have supplementary calcium.

Table 9.2. Major dietary sources of calcium (approximate values)

Nutrient	Calcium mg/100g
Primary food sources of calcium	
Milk, whole	111
Milk, skimmed	124
Yoghurt	134
Cheese	600--1,000
Ice cream	120
Secondary food sources of calcium	
Beans	65
Nuts	75
Almonds	250
Salmon, canned with bones	200
Sardines, canned with bones	300
Broccoli, cooked	130
Spinach, cooked	160
Rhubarb, cooked	300
Kale, cooked	200
Parsley	100

Adapted from Charles [A24]

Low fat cheeses are especially recommended. Moreover, lactose in milk facilitates absorption of calcium by the gut.

▶ *Fresh, green vegetables, fruits, and wheat products* are important sources of calcium. However, it should be pointed out that oxalate in some vegetables inhibits its absorption. Wheat products are also good sources of calcium, except for white bread and some other processed varieties. Likewise, addition of sugar, salt, phosphate, fat, and protein can substantially decrease calcium absorption (see below).

▶ *Mineral water*: This can contribute to a positive calcium balance when the water is enriched with calcium. But the amount in each type of mineral water varies and may range from 10 to 650 mg/l. The exact amount is always stated on the label on the bottle.

Fortified juices may solve the calcium dilemma in patients who cannot eat dairy products because of allergies.

▶ *Fruit juices*: These are particularly useful for patients with allergies to milk or milk products, especially if they have been fortified by addition of calcium. Moreover, the vitamin D in the fruit juice increases absorption of calcium from 30 % (milk and milk products) to 40 %. Addition of vitamin D may further increase intestinal absorption of calcium.

Calcium tablets. Additional calcium in the form of tablets should only be taken on medical advice. There are some dangers if excessive amounts of calcium are taken, including the possibility of kidney stones. Only some 200 mg calcium are absorbed when 500 mg calcium carbonate is taken. Calcium citrate has been found to dissolve more easily than carbonate, phosphate, lactate, or gluconate, and is about 60% more bioavailable in the body. While calcium carbonate and calcium phosphate must be taken with food, because gastric acid is required for absorption, calcium citrate can be taken with or without food. It also has the advantage of not producing gas or causing constipation, but it is more expensive. The following hints may help to get the maximum benefit from calcium tablets:

▶ A single dose should not exceed 500 mg, so the daily amount should be taken in divided doses as necessary.
▶ One dose before bedtime inhibits loss of bone during the night.
▶ Calcium should be taken with meals. Absorption in the gut is also improved by vitamin C as well as a little fat and protein together with the tablets.
▶ Absorption is inhibited by foods rich in fibres and in fat.
▶ Calcium should not be taken together with iron as these combine to form insoluble compounds and so are lost to the body.

Other useful minerals. Numerous minerals are necessary for absorption of calcium including magnesium, boron, copper, manganese, zinc, silicon, strontium, fluoride, and phosphorus. They are also essential for normal growth of bones and play an important role in bone metabolism and turnover. The best way to ensure the correct balance is through a variety of foods, as these minerals may be dangerous if taken in too large amounts. *Magnesium* especially is essential for bone health:

▶ Activates osteoblasts
▶ Increases mineralisation density
▶ Activates vitamin D
▶ Enhances sensitivity of bone tissue to PTH and active vitamin D
▶ Facilitates the transport of calcium in and out of bone

About 60% of magnesium is stored in bone, followed by muscles and other tissues. The recommended dosages are 300–500 mg, with an ap-

Bone-building nutrients, also called "bone boosters".

Other nutrients such as magnesium and vitamin K are also important to bone health. Make sure to include all substances required for skeletal health.

propriate calcium/magnesium ratio of 2:1. Since high single doses of magnesium may cause diarrhoea, it is best to distribute the total amount throughout the day. However, there is little evidence that magnesium is needed to prevent osteoporosis in the general population.

Step 2: An Adequate Supply of Vitamins

Calcium and vitamin D intake maximises the efficacy of other osteoporosis therapies.

Vitamin D promotes bone formation by improving intestinal absorption of calcium and phosphate and by stimulating maturation and mineralisation of the osseous ground substance – the osteoid. A daily allowance of 400–800 IU is required for healthy bone. A daily 15-min sunbath would be required for an individual to produce an equal quantity of vitamin D. However, today's living conditions, the use of sun filter creams, and the fear of skin cancer all combine to rule out the possibility of adequate production of vitamin D by the skin. In addition, the conversion of sunlight into vitamin D in older people is only half that of younger people. Consequently, a daily intake of 800–1,000 IU of vitamin D in the form of tablets with meals is reasonable and cost-effective.

Vitamins: plentiful in fresh fruits and vegetables, but most people don't get enough without additional supplements – so don't forget to take them.

Vitamin C, another new player in bone health, is required for maturation of collagen (crosslinking); it stimulates the bone-forming cells (osteoblasts) and improves absorption of calcium. 60 mg vitamin C is the minimal daily requirement, enough to prevent scurvy, but not enough to reap all the possible benefits. The best sources are citrus fruits. Ideally, 1,000 mg should be taken as calcium ascorbate. Epidemiologic studies have shown a positive association between vitamin C and bone mass.

Vitamin K is now recognised as a "new" bone-building vitamin. Though better known for its part in coagulation, it plays a significant role in synthesis of osteocalcin, one of the building blocks of bone. Vitamin K mediates the attachment of calcium to bone matrix and is also required for fracture healing. Observational studies have shown that women with higher intake and serum levels of vitamin K tend to have higher bone densities, and patients who sustain fractures have been reported to have lower serum vitamin K levels. 100–300 µg vitamin K are required daily, taken with meals. It is produced by bacteria normally found in the intestinal tract (menaquinone). Dark-green vegetables (e. g., spinach or broccoli) also contain large amounts of vitamin K (phylloquinone). Since this is a fat-soluble vitamin, it is helpful to consume vitamin K-rich foods with a little fat or oil.

Vitamin A is a fat-soluble vitamin and so can be stored by the body. It influences the development of bone cells. The recommended daily allowance is 5,000 IU.

Vitamin B_{12} and folic acid are necessary for formation as well as maintenance of healthy bones. Vitamin B_{12} protects the bones against the effects of homocysteine, and the levels decrease with age. The recommended daily dose of vitamin B_{12} is 1 mg.

Step 3: Protect the Spine in Everyday Living

Thoracic and lumbar vertebrae are composed largely of cancellous bone and therefore highly susceptible to fracture – due to the combined effects of trabecular bone loss and weight bearing. Osteoporosis usually starts with collapse of the upper and lower plates of the vertebrae and protrusion into the vertebral bodies. When the BMD shows osteoporotic values, everyday life should be adapted to ensure protection for the spine and hip joints:

A strong back is vital to skeleton strength.

▶ *Activity while upright*: upright posture in front of a working surface adapted to the height of the worker.
▶ *Activity while sitting*: The back of the chair should provide support for the spine from 15–12 cm above the seat of the chair. The spine should not be curved (danger of wedge fractures!). One should never stay for long in the sitting position but every now and then get up, stretch, and move around.
▶ *Load lifting and carrying*: Do not bend down with a curved back and straight legs! This may damage the lumbar discs and cause vertebral body compression. Rather bend the knees, lift up the load, and rise up keeping the spine straight. This applies especially to heavy objects such as cartons of drinks.
▶ *Housework*: During the daily performance of household activities bending or curving the spine should be avoided, better to go down on one's knees or to crouch.
▶ *Lying down and sleeping*: Soft mattresses should be avoided, but a flexible mattress on a hard frame is recommended as it gives equal support to the whole body. Also recommended is a small flat pillow, just to provide support for the head and neck.

Fractures do not have to happen! And it is never too late for fracture prevention.

Fig. 9.1. Upright posture: head held high, shoulders back, and tummy in assure proper alignment and good posture

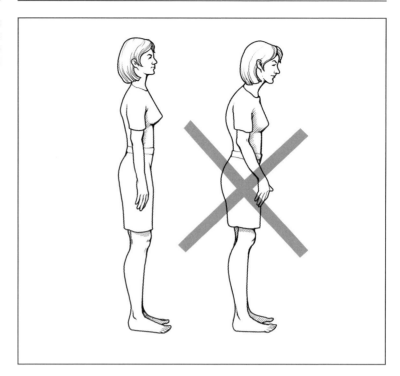

Fig. 9.2. Proper sitting: sitting upright with feet on the floor reduces stress on the spine

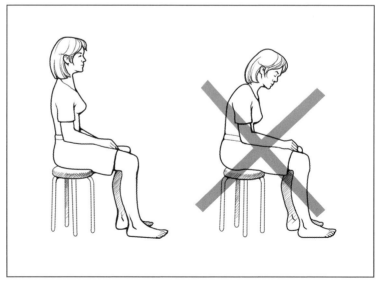

Table 9.3. Guidelines for safe movement for osteoporotic patients

- Proper posture and alignment when standing, sitting or walking: lift breastbone, keep head erect, look forward, keep shoulders back, gently tighten abdominal muscles, maintain small hollow in the lower back.
- Standing for a long time: point feet straight ahead, periodically switch from one foot to the other.
- Sitting: use a pillow at the small of the back, maintain upright alignment, rest feet flat on the floor or on a small footstool. Sit on chairs with backs, not on stools.
- Standing from a chair: move hips forward to front of the chair, shift weight over the feet leading with a lifted chest, stand by pushing down into the floor using leg muscles, the arm muscles can assist by pushing down on arm rests of the chair.
- Walking: hold chin in and head upright, point feet straight ahead.
- Bending: keep feet shoulder width apart, maintain straight back, bend at the hips and knees (not the waist), avoid twisting and bending together, use one hand on a stable support devise.
- Lifting: keep object close to the body, first kneel on one knee and stand with the object close to the waist, use lightly packed plastic grocery packages with handles and carry one in each hand. Following acute vertebral fracture, limit weight to 4.5 kg.
- Tying shoes: first, sit in a chair, cross one foot over the opposite knee or rest one foot on a stool.
- Getting in and out bed: in – sit on the edge of the bed, lean trunk towards head of bed and lower body down with the help of one arm, while lowering trunk to the bed, bring legs and feet on to the bed, roll on to the back with knees bent; reverse for getting out of bed.
- Coughing and sneezing: gently tighten abdominal muscles to support back, and place one hand on the back, or press back into chair or wall for support.

From "Boning Up On Osteoporosis: A Guide to Prevention and Treatment." Washington DC National Osteoporosis Foundation, 2003

Step 4: Regular Physical Activity

Bone, muscles, and joints are all strengthened by movement. The theory that putting stress or forces of gravity onto the skeletal system causes it to form more bone is known as *Wolff's law*. Physical fitness ensures confidence both in locomotion and coordination. Physical activity stimulates blood flow and stabilises blood pressure, which in turn decreases attacks of dizziness in older people, a common cause of falling. In the event of a fracture anybody who exercises regularly will have shorter periods of pain as well as of recovery. Training and exercise should be regular rather than irregular and then exaggerated. Comparative studies have shown that women who walk daily for half an hour have stronger bones than those who do not.

Stop saying "I am too old to exercise!" Everybody can exercise in some form, and age is not a limiting factor. But you must be active every day without fail.

The optimal exercise regimen for preventing osteoporosis and related fractures is not known. A recent Swedish study of randomly selected elderly women could not confirm an effect of previous and present everyday physical activity on bone mass. However, any exer-

Your exercise program should take place in a group and should be fun.

cise is better than none, and consistent activity is associated with the greatest long-term benefit. Indeed, current or past activity is associated with a 20%–60% reduction in the rate of hip fractures in both women and men. Weight-bearing exercises which work against gravity such as climbing mountains or stairs (instead of the elevator) and walking, running, and jumping are the most effective in strengthening the bones. Drive the car only when absolutely necessary! Moreover, regular sport – in one form or another – improves the quality of life. However, it must be stated that if the person concerned does not enjoy a particular activity it won't be carried out regularly – if at all – and therefore the exercise sport or activity chosen must be in tune with the patients' wishes and abilities. In addition, it is advisable to choose a sport or activity which involves as many muscle groups as possible, as well as not causing physical complaints and pain. Today, sport-oriented institutions and clubs offer a whole variety of activities in a friendly and social environment. There are no age limits. For sedentary or frail elderly, a program of walking, low-impact aerobics or light gardening in addition to a muscle strengthening program is recommended. Training-induced gains in strength are initially rapid but tend to plateau after more than 12 weeks, even with progressive increases in training loads. When correlating mechanical load with bone mass, there is greater gain in bone mass at the lowest levels of activity (complete immobility to sedentary) than at the highest (moderately active to walking with high impact loading).

Anything that works your muscles against your bones causes bone growth and strength.

It has been shown that in *childhood and adolescence* bone responds more favourably to mechanical loading than at other ages. It was shown in a study with female tennis players that when training was begun before menarche, differences in bone mineral density in the humerus ranged from 17% to 24% compared to 8% to 14% when training began after menarche. In 15–20 year-old Olympic weightlifters, the mean distal and proximal forearm BMD was 51% and 41% above the age-matched controls, respectively. Swimming, on the other hand, did not increase bone mass as measured by DXA. Although elite swimmers undertake intense training programs, their BMD was similar to that of control subjects. There is some evidence that higher levels of bone attained in childhood are maintained in gymnasts. Whether childhood physical activity, however, influences the rate or timing of adult bone loss is not known. It should be pointed out that there is a peak fracture incidence in young people – 10–14 years in girls and 15–19 years in boys. These fractures are not related to osteoporosis, but

Get 30 min of weight-bearing exercise three to five times a week.

are the result of falls or trauma sustained during intense physical activity – possibly "extreme sports." These are completely healthy, well-nourished young people with no deficiencies whatever.

More attention must be devoted to the role of exercise for *osteoporotic patients* or those who have already sustained fractures. Usually these patients show reluctance to participate in an exercise program because they may have pain or fear of additional fractures. However, avoidance of any activity will aggravate further bone loss. Bed-bound bones rapidly lose bone mass, and a bed-rest study showed that trabecular bone was lost at a rate of about 1% per week and cortical bone at a rate of about 1% per month. Restoration of bone mass is much slower than bone loss: about 1% per month for trabecular bone. An exercise program should increase the ability to carry out routine daily activities while minimizing the risk of falls or subsequent fractures. Patients with vertebral fractures should avoid activities that place an anterior load on vertebral bodies, such as back flexion exercise. When advising patients with osteoarthritis or associated conditions, patients who have been previously sedentary and frail, elderly patients, physicians should consider referring the patients to physical therapists to start with a moderate exercise program and for instruction in proper exercise techniques. Patients with cardiovascular diseases require cardiologic consultation for risk evaluation before starting an exercise program.

A few precautions for runners: Wear good running shoes, run on soft surfaces and take shorter strides.

Step 5: No Smoking

Every smoker has the power – in the truest sense of the word – to stop smoking and thereby reduce by half the risk of osteoporosis. Smokers have almost double the risk of hip fractures compared to nonsmokers. Up to 20% of all hip fractures are attributed to cigarette smoking. Women who smoke a pack a day have 10% less mineral bone density at the menopause than nonsmokers. Studies have shown that smokers sustain fractures of the vertebral bodies earlier and more frequently than nonsmokers, while fracture-healing is delayed or prolonged (or both). Smokers also experience menopause one or two years earlier than nonsmokers.

Four risk factors are key determinants for risk of hip fracture:
- Personal history of fracture
- Family history of fracture
- Smoking
- Low body weight

Smoking produces a number of *effects* harmful to bone:
▶ Decreases production of oestrogen in women

▶ Increases breakdown of oestrogen in the liver
▶ Decreases production of testosterone in men
▶ Reduces conversion of adrenal androgens to oestrogens
▶ Damages bone and bone cells by means of many toxic substances
▶ Decreases blood-flow through bone and bone marrow circulations
▶ Effects pulmonary function and causes decreased uptake of oxygen
▶ Creates free radicals

Some experts are convinced that the anti-oestrogen effects of smoking are enough to cancel the effects of oestrogen therapy in the menopause. In men, smoking causes a significant reduction in testosterone levels which (as in women) results in decreased mineral bone density, i.e. accelerated loss of bone. This loss occurs primarily in trabecular bone and particularly in the vertebral bodies of the spine. Moreover, smokers harbour a higher concentration of substances harmful to bone: these include cadmium, lead, and other toxic substances. It should be noted that today there are many successful programs and strategies available to help people to stop smoking.

Step 6: Reduce Nutritional "Bone Robbers"

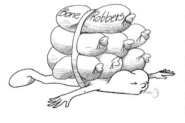

These are substances in food that require calcium for their metabolism, neutralisation, and elimination. These substances are usually not recognised as damaging, which enables them to withdraw calcium from bone and thereby increase bone loss unobserved. *Bone robbers* include the following:

Moderate intake of alcohol may even slightly improve bone density and decrease fracture risk.

High alcohol intake. This inhibits absorption of important building-blocks for bone and damages the liver, an organ required for activation of vitamin D. Moreover, manifest hepatic cirrhosis also causes malabsorption by reducing the flow of bile. In addition, alcohol damages the bone cells directly. Many male alcoholics suffer from androgen deficiency, which in turn aggravates osteoporosis. Alcohol also has a negative effect on the immature skeleton. In contrast, small quantities have been shown to have a beneficial effect on bone in older women.

Caffeine. Caffeine acts as a diuretic, causing an increased urinary excretion of calcium and magnesium. People with a low calcium intake

Table 9.4. Effects of nutrients on calcium metabolism

Nutrients	Increase in urine calcium	Decrease in calcium absorption
High protein	X	
High salt	X	
High phosphorus	X	
High sugar	X	
Vitamin D deficiency		X
Oxalates (rhubarb, spinach)		X
Phytates (wheat, bran, beans)		X
Iron		X
High caffeine (>4 cups daily)	X	X

are especially vulnerable to this loss. Patients who do not – for one reason or another – limit their consumption of coffee are advised to drink a glass of milk for each cup of coffee to restore the calcium balance. It would be prudent to avoid excessive intake (>4 cups of coffee per day) and to make sure that calcium intake is sufficient, i.e., to make up for the loss. Phosphate is the culprit in drinks made with cola, because the high content of phosphate binds calcium in the gut and thereby reduces its absorption. Many medicines, including aspirin and other pain relievers, diet aids, and diuretics also have caffeine as an ingredient. On the other hand, tea – though also a caffeine-containing drink – is associated with a decrease in femoral neck fractures possibly because tea contains flavinoids.

Drinking one cup of milk per cup of coffee helps offset the negative calcium balance.

Sugar. Consumption of sugar has increased 1,000-fold during the past 100 years. About half of the intake of carbohydrates consists of sugar. Furthermore, the metabolism of sugar in the body utilises vitamins and augments the renal excretion of valuable substances such as calcium, magnesium, and other minerals. In addition, sugar also inhibits uptake of calcium in the intestines as well as stimulating the secretion of acids in the stomach – another "bone robber." In particular, the combination of coffee and sugar, as in very sweet black strong coffee or in "soft drinks" such as Coca Cola is a veritable "bone gobbler." Consequently, it is not surprising that healthy teeth and strong bones are characteristic of countries with a low overall consumption of sugar.

Life as a whole will be "sweeter" when consumption of sugar and sweets is reduced.

The sodium/calcium connection: Salt intake plays an important role in determining blood pressure and bone density.

Salt. It has long been established that a high intake of salt is associated with an increased risk of high blood pressure and its associated disorders. In contrast to patients with normal blood pressure, hypertensives have a higher loss of calcium in the urine with its attendant risk of osteoporosis. In addition, some people seem to be more sensitive to the effects of salts than others. A sodium intake of less than 2,400 mg/day is recommended. Every additional 500 mg of salt takes another 10 mg of calcium out of the bones, because sodium competes with calcium for reabsorption in the renal tubules. The latest studies have shown that limiting salt intake is directly associated with a decreased risk of osteoporosis.

Proteins. Acids, especially phosphoric and sulfuric acids, are produced during the metabolism and breakdown of proteins. These acids must first be neutralised – buffered – by combining with calcium before they are eliminated by the kidneys; otherwise the body would be "acidified." Meat protein is more acidic during digestion than protein from fish, diary products, beans, nuts, and seeds because these consist of different amino acids and different kinds of fatty acids. When protein intake is high while that of calcium is low, a "negative calcium balance" is created and the required calcium is mobilised from the bones. So, avoiding excessive protein intakes (>60 g/d) will improve calcium balance and overall health. Vegetarians with their low consumption of animal proteins always show a positive calcium balance and stable bones. On the other hand, Eskimos with their high intake of animal protein and low consumption of calcium suffer a 20 % greater loss of bone than Europeans.

Phosphate. Combined with calcium it produces a strong crystalline substance which gives teeth and bones their hardness. Ideally, one part phosphate should combine with one part calcium. However, our diet contains far more phosphate than is required. This in turn triggers secretion of parathormone to neutralise the excess phosphate by mobilisation of calcium and magnesium from the bones. Meat products, soft drinks, and many prepared "ready-to eat" and "fast foods" contain high levels of phosphate and their intake should be correspondingly restricted.

Lipids. Prior to absorption into the blood stream calcium is dissolved in the acidic gastric juices and combined with lipids. Only in this form can calcium be taken up by the gastric mucosa and pass into the circulation. But when too much fat is present, the opposite effect occurs – calcium and magnesium are lost and bone is lost too. The deleterious effect of fat on bone is illustrated by comparison of the incidence of osteoporosis in the "low-lipid countries" of the Far East, with that of the USA, where it is significantly higher.

Over-acidification. In actual fact, our bodies are swamped by acids produced by the body itself or absorbed with food (proteins, sugars, fats) in large quantities. The acids have to be neutralised, and this is accomplished in the skeleton. The bones harbour a large quantity of alkaline salts such as calcium, potassium, sodium, and magnesium which are mobilised immediately to neutralise any acids in the blood. The connection between an acidic pH-value and osteoporosis is well-known and is taken into consideration in any program for prevention of osteoporosis. These observations underline the importance of sufficient quantities of basic vegetables and fruits in order to supply the body with these alkaline substances as well as with vitamins. It is clear therefore that vegetables and fruits are required for neutralisation of acids and milk and its products for an adequate supply of calcium.

Step 7: An Ideal Body Weight

All large osteoporosis studies have demonstrated the close connection between osteoporosis and low body weight. Underweight individuals consume insufficient calories and insufficient materials to maintain their bodies. A low body weight and a low muscle mass result in less stimulation of the bones, hence lower bone mass. Women with less body fat also tend to produce less oestrogen. However, obesity should not be encouraged because of its many harmful effects on health. The best course is to aim for a weight that is normal for height and body build.

A successful bone-building programme must include also mind and body concepts!

Step 8: Drugs that Cause Osteoporosis

A comprehensive list of drugs associated with increased risk of osteoporosis in adults has been outlined by the National Osteoporosis

Foundation. The most commonly used groups of drugs are given in Chapter 22.

Glucocorticoids. Exogenous glucocorticoid excess is the most frequent cause of secondary osteoporosis. This group includes all substances derived from cortisone, such as prednisone and dexamethasone. Bone loss may be rapid, particularly in children and in women over 50 years. The BMD should be measured in all patients before starting long-term therapy with glucocorticoids, and subsequently every six months thereafter for the course of the treatment. Patients with low bone mass or even fractures should be considered for therapy with antiresorptive agents. However, short-term local application of cortisone derivatives such as ointments or sprays are not damaging to bone. Not all patients experience the same degree of bone loss even with the same or similar medications. Two major factors influence bone loss: the quantity and the length of the period during which the medication is taken. Therefore, the daily dose and the period of administration should be kept to a minimum. When prednisone is unavoidable the patient should be advised to stop smoking, to take calcium and vitamin D tablets, and to undertake regular sport or other physical activity.

Thyroid hormones. They have two applications: to prevent development of struma and to treat hypothyroidism. Overdosage, which might occur with prolonged administration, should be avoided, as this may also lead to osteoporosis and fractures.

Anticoagulants. Heparin and warfarin given over long periods (years) may cause severe osteoporosis.

Anticonvulsants. These include carbamazepine, phenytoin, and barbiturates. They can damage bone over time and cause disturbances in mineralisation as well as bone loss ("osteoporomalacia").

Many *other medications* also weaken the bones on prolonged use. This list includes: antidepressives, lithium, antibiotics, isoniazide, antacids containing aluminium, and cytostatic drugs. Any medication taken by a patient should be checked for its potential to effect bone adversely so that precautions may be taken in advance.

Step 9: Diseases that Damage Bones

Primary chronic polyarthritis (PCP) is probably the most important representative of this group. Over the years PCP has consistently caused osteoporosis and fractures. Damage to bones is further aggravated by three additional factors: patients are treated with corticoids, they are limited in their movements, and they are underweight.

Chronic pulmonary diseases, especially bronchitis and emphysema caused by smoking, increase the risk of osteoporosis, which is further enhanced by the drugs often given as therapy.

Chronic cardiac insufficiency. This leads to increased resorption of bone because of limitations in mobility and secondary hyperparathyroidism. Consequently, when a heart transplant is considered, it is advisable to institute bisphosphonate therapy months in advance to avert the otherwise inevitable loss of bone.

Diabetes mellitus. This in itself constitutes a considerable risk for osteoporosis. The lack of insulin causes an increase in bone resorption as well as a decrease in production of collagen. This effects mainly patients who are treated with tablets.

Inflammatory bowel disorders and gastric/intestinal operations. A decrease in absorption of calcium and vitamin D is characteristic. In these cases, particular attention must be paid to an adequate diet and sufficient vitamin intake.

Renal insufficiency. The pathogenesis of renal bone disease is complex, multifactorial, and incompletely understood. This disease is dealt with in Chap. 21.

Exercise is perhaps the most powerful medicine available to us.

Table 9.5. Recommendations of NOF's physician's Guide to prevention and treatment of osteoporosis

- Counsel women on the risk factors for osteoporosis.
- Evaluate for osteoporosis in all postmenopausal women presenting with fractures and confirm a positive diagnosis with a bone mineral density (BMD) test.
- Recommend BMD assessment for postmenopausal women under age 65 years with one or more additional risk factors (fractures, low body weight, smokers).
- Recommend BMD assessment for postmenopausal women over age 65 years.
- Advise all patients to obtain adequate dietary calcium (at least 1,200 mg/day, including supplements if necessary) and vitamin D (400–800 IU/day for individuals at risk of deficiency).
- Advise patients to avoid tobacco use and to keep alcohol intake moderate (two drinks or fewer per day).
- Consider all patients who present with vertebral or hip fractures to be candidates for treatment of osteoporosis.
- Initiate therapy to reduce fracture risk in patients with low BMD.
- Patients over age 70 years with multiple risk factors (especially those with previous nonhip, nonspine fractures) are at sufficiently high risk for osteoporosis that treatment is warranted without BMD testing. BMD measurement can be used to establish or confirm a diagnosis of osteoporosis, predict future fracture risk, and monitor changes in BMD due to medical conditions or therapy.
- Pharmacological options include: bisphosphonates, such as alendronate and risedronate, calcitonin, oestrogen or hormone therapy (ET/HT), parathyroid hormone, and a selective oestrogen receptor modulator (SERM), raloxifene.

National Osteoporosis Foundation (NOF) 2003

Evidence-Based Medicine for Therapy of Osteoporosis

The major aim of therapy is prevention of fractures. It should be pointed out right away that there are considerable differences in both quality and credibility in results of randomised trials dealing with efficacy of various treatment schedules. When results of these clinical trials are assessed and compared, problems arise with respect to the following criteria:

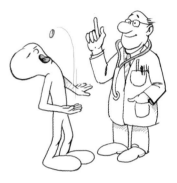

► Duration of the study
► Number and age of the patients
► Definition of exclusion criteria
► Primary aim of the study
► Fracture incidence versus fracture rate
► Fractures prior to start of study
► Definition of "fracture"
► Definition of "control group"
► Status of vitamin D and calcium
► Method and accuracy of bone density measurements
► Differences in statistics used for analysis

It is now possible to evaluate results of studies and reports of experiences in an objective and balanced fashion ("*evidence-based medicine*") especially with reference to

► Meta-analysis of randomised controlled trials (RCTs)
► Individual randomised controlled studies
► Studies based on observations
► Results of basic research
► Results and reports of clinical experience

Just as treatment is now available to control hypertension and high blood cholesterol, treatment is also available to control osteoporosis and fractures.

Table 10.1. Large RCTs of antiresorptive therapies with fracture as an endpoint in postmenopausal women with osteoporosis

Agent	Study	First author, year	Patients (n)	Duration
Alendronate	FIT 1	Black 1996 [7]	2,027 1,022/1,005 ALN/PLA	3 years
	FIT 2	Cummings 1998 [15]	4,432 2,214/2,218 ALN/PLA	4 years
	FOSIT	Pols 1999 [35]	1,908 950/958 ALN/PLA	1 year
	Liberman	Liberman 1995 [26]	994 526/355 ALN/PLA	8 years
Risedronate	VERT-NA	Harris 1999 [22]	2,458 813/815 RIS/PLA	3 years
	VERT-MN	Reginster 2000 [37]	1,226 407/407 RIS/PLA	3 years
	HIP	McClung 2001 [31]	9,331	3 years
			5,445 1,812/1,821 RIS/PLA 3,886 1,292/1,313 RIS/PLA	
Raloxifene	MORE	Ettinger 1999 [19]	7,705 5,129/2,576 RAL/PLA	3 years
	MORE 1		3,002/1,522 RAL/PLA	
	MORE 2		1,534/770 RAL/PLA	
Calcitonin	PROOF	Chesnut 2000 [14]	1,255 CAL/PLA	5 years

ALN, alendronate; *CAL*, salmon calcitonin; *RIS*, risedronate; *RAL*, raloxifene; *PLA*, placebo; *Vert.Fx*, vertebral fractures; *HipFx*, hip fractures; *NonVert.Fx*, nonvertebral fractures; *Clin.Fx*, clinical fractures; *BMD*, bone mineral density of the lumbar spine

Primary endpoint	Completers	Age, mean	Prevalent Vert.Fx
Vert.Fx –20 %/4mm	89 % ALA 87 % PLA	55–81 71	0 %
Clin.Fx –20 %/4mm	4,272 96 % 93 % ALA 94 % PLA	54–81 68	0 %
BMD	?	–85 63	?
Vert.Fx –20 %/4mm	89 %	45–80 64	18 %
Vert.Fx –15 %	55 % PLA 60 % RIS	–85 69	80 %
Vert.Fx –15 %	54 % PLA 62 % RIS	–85 71	98 %
HipFx Secondary: NonVert.Fx, BMD	64 %		18 % total 31 % group 1
	57 % RIS 57 % PLA	70–79	
	41 % RIS 42 % PLA	>80	
Vert.Fx –20 %/4 mm, BMD Secondary: NonVert.Fx	89 % 79 % RAL 75 % PLA	31–80 67	
		65	11 %
		68/69	89 %
Vert.Fx Secondary: Nonvert.Fx	41 %	68	79 %

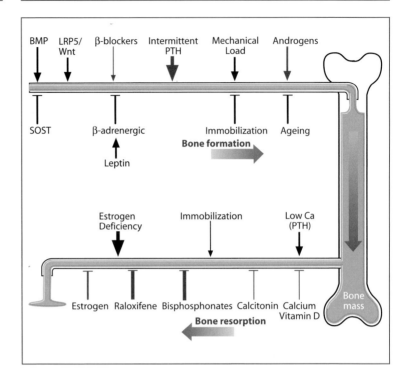

Fig. 10.1. Physiological factors and therapeutic agents and their influence on bone remodelling and bone mass. Physiological (*black*) and pharmacological (*red*) stimulators and inhibitors of bone formation and resorption are listed. The relative impact, where known, is represented by the thickness of the arrows. *BMP*, bone morphogenetic proteins; *SOST*, sclerostin; *LRP5*, low density lipoprotein (LDL)-receptor-related protein; *PTH*, parathyroid hormone; *SERM*, selective oestrogen-receptor modulator. (Modified from Harada and Rodan [A61])

With the continuing world-wide acceptance of evidence-based methodology, the classification of levels of evidence and the grading of recommendations are becoming better known and are the basis of an effective and rational treatment of osteoporosis:

Levels of Evidence

Ia   From meta-analysis of randomised controlled trials (RCTs)

Ib   From at least one large RCT

IIa From at least one well-designed controlled study without randomisation

IIb From at least one other type of well-designed quasiexperimental study

III From well-designed, nonexperimental descriptive studies

IV From expert committee reports or opinions

Grading of Recommendations

A Levels Ia and Ib

B Levels IIa, IIb, and III

C Level IV

When this rigorous approach of evidence-based medicine is adopted, the most conclusive evidence for reducing fracture risk (*"A class" recommendation*) has been shown for:

▶ Supplements with calcium and vitamin D
▶ Therapy with alendronate or risedronate
▶ Therapy with raloxifen (SERM)
▶ Therapy with parathormone (PTH)

These five A-recommended drugs/substances should have first priority in osteoporosis therapy. In contrast, no reliable or definite data are available as yet for calcitonin, etidronate, fluoride, and calcitriol so no conclusions could be drawn as to fracture risk. Thus, it has now been conclusively shown that the N-containing bisphosphonates (e. g. alendronate and risedronate) achieve the greatest reduction in fracture risk: on average a 50 % reduction in vertebral and extravertebral fractures after one year of therapy.

The concept of a placebo-controlled trial has been challenged on the basis that it is no longer ethical to place osteoporotic patients on placebo now that proven effective therapies are available. New recommendations have been suggested but as yet no official decisions have been taken. However, in a paper published by the Center for Medical

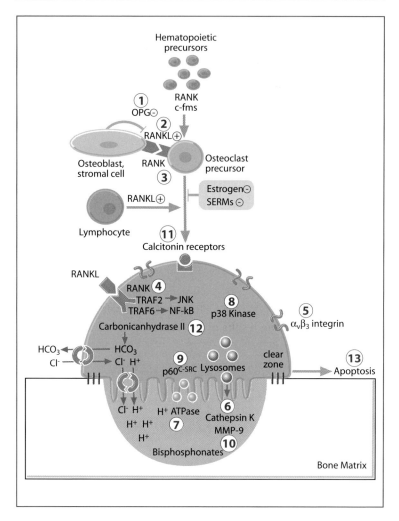

Fig. 10.2. Diagram of development and activation of the osteoclast illustrating points of potential therapeutic targets indicated by numbers. (Modified from Rodan and Martin [A118])

Ethics and Health Policy (June 2003), the conclusion is reached that "if placebo controls put subjects at substantial risk of serious outcomes they are not ethically permissible." The FDA's Osteoporotic Guidance document has recently been revised (June 2003) and directions for future developments provided.

Comprehensive Approach to Therapy of Osteoporosis

Successful therapy of osteoporosis includes the following aspects:

▶ Treatment of pain
▶ Initiation of physical activity and exercises
▶ Prevention of falls
▶ Adaptation of life-style for skeletal health
▶ Bone-conscious nutrition
▶ Vitamin D and calcium supplements
▶ Hormone replacement therapy (HRT) for short periods only! Or substitutes
▶ Antiresorptive therapy (bisphophonates, raloxifene, calcitonin)
▶ Osteoanabolic therapy (fluoride, strontium, anabolics, parathormone)
▶ Other medications (statins, growth factors, tetracyclins, leptin)

The individual components of the therapeutic spectrum given above must be tailored to the special needs and requirements of each patient. However, based on the results of the evidence-based medicine cited above, the following *treatment strategy* is employed in our out-patient clinic:

It is never too early and never too late to battle osteoporosis!

▶ All patients are given vitamin D and calcium supplements
▶ HRT or its equivalent is discussed with each female patient, but is no longer advocated for treatment of osteoporosis alone
▶ Early administration of a modern (nitrogen-containing) bisphosphonate
▶ Early administration of raloxifen

In summary: several excellent reviews on osteoporosis have been published. It is noteworthy that osteoporosis is a global condition and that similar approaches and guidelines on osteoporosis have been recommended in many countries including Australia, Brazil, Canada, European Union, India, Japan, and the USA (in alphabetical order).

Table 10.2. Medications used in osteoporosis

US FDA-approved medications for osteoporosis

- Alendronate (Brand name: Fosamax): Alendronate is approved by the FDA for the prevention and treatment of postmenopausal osteoporosis (10 mg daily or 70 mg weekly). Alendronate is also approved as a treatment in men with osteoporosis, additionally it is approved for the treatment of osteoporosis in both men and women as a result of prolonged glucocorticoid use. Alendronate, in a 5 mg daily dose or 35 mg weekly dose, is been approved by the FDA for prevention of postmenopausal osteoporosis.
- Risedronate (Brand name: Actonel): Risedronate, 5 mg daily or 35 mg weekly, is approved by the FDA for the prevention and treatment of postmenopausal osteoporosis. It is also approved for the prevention and treatment of glucocorticoid-induced osteoporosis.
- Raloxifene (Brand name: Evista, Optruma): Raloxifene is approved by the FDA for both prevention and treatment of postmenopausal osteoporosis.
- Parathyroid hormone – teriparatide or PTH (1–34) (Brand name: Fortéo): Teriparatide is an injectable form of human parathyroid hormone that is approved by the FDA for the treatment of osteoporosis in postmenopausal women and men who are at high risk for having a fracture.
- Calcitonin (Brand name: Miacalcin, Karil, and others): Salmon calcitonin is approved by the FDA for the treatment of osteoporosis in women who are at least five years postmenopausal.
- Oestrogen/Hormone Therapy (ET/HT) (Brand name: Climare, Estraderm, and others, Activella, and others): ET/HT therapy is approved by the FDA for the prevention of osteoporosis, relief of vasomotor symptoms and vulvovaginal atrophy associated with menopause. The FDA recommends that when ET/HT use is considered solely for prevention of osteoporosis, other approved nonoestrogen treatments should first be carefully considered.

US FDA-nonapproved medications for osteoporosis

- Other bisphophonates (etidronate, tiludronate, pamidronate, ibandronate, zoledronate): At the time of publication, none have been approved for prevention or treatment of osteoporosis in the USA. However, several are approved for use outside the USA. These medications are currently approved for a variety of bone disorders. Ibandronate, a potent bisphosphonate, can be given either intravenously or orally, and zoledronate, given intravenously, are under evaluation as treatment of osteoporosis.
- Calcitriol: It has been approved by the FDA only for managing hypocalcemia and metabolic bone disease in renal dialysis patients.
- Fluoride: The evidence that fluoride reduces fracture risk is conflicting and controversial.
- Tibolone: This oestrogen-like agent is prescribed in Europe for the treatment of vasomotor symptoms of menopause, but has not been approved for use in the USA.

Adapted from F. Bonner Jr. et al. [A13]

Treat the Patient, Not Only the Disease

Osteoporotic pain is usually acute, of sudden onset, and caused by a fracture in the lower thoracic or lumbar vertebrae. On examination, there will be a painful spot in the area of the back where the vertebral fracture has occurred. The muscles next to the spine will be very tense and painful to touch. This pain can last for long periods ranging from a few weeks to months. In all patients, an X-ray of the affected skeletal area should be taken to demonstrate or rule out a vertebral fracture and to document the extent of destruction of bone. A bone scan may demonstrate an acute inflammation around an area of fractured bone and may therefore show fractured vertebrae long before a regular X-ray because of the increased uptake in that area. It has further been suggested that covert small fractures – microfractures – due to mechanical stress can also cause pain. When the intraosseous pressure exceeds a certain level, fluid in the bone enters the subperiosteal space, exercises pressure on the nerves, and induces a painful periosteal reaction. Pain during healing of a fracture may well be related to local release of cytokines, prostanoids, histamine, and bradykinin in the surrounding area.

Pain is one of the most difficult problems associated with osteoporosis. But inadequate pain management is no longer acceptable under any circumstances.

Acute Phase

For immediate treatment of *acute pain*, peripherally active analgetics are generally administered first. These include acetylsalicylic acid, paracetamol, metamizol, and especially nonsteroidal antirheumatic drugs, which act by local inhibition of prostaglandins. But these should only be taken for short periods of time because of their possible harmful effects on the gastric mucosa and on the bone marrow.

The simplest measure of the intensity of acute pain is a visual analogue scale.

Never despair! If one set
of measures doesn't work –
another will!

However, the latest in this series of antirheumatic drugs such as COX-2-inhibitor do not have these side effects. Bone pain can also be rapidly and effectively treated with bisphosphonates, which have largely replaced calcitonin for this purpose. When the pain is very strong, as in a recent fracture, the medications listed above can be combined with a weak opiate. If the treatment outlined above is not enough, a pain expert can be consulted and the treatment adjusted according to the advice given. It is advisable to avoid muscle relaxants as they increase the risk of falling because of their sedative action. Bed rest is recommended for the acute stage but only until the acute pain has subsided. Subsequently, short periods of careful weight bearing alternating with exercises are incorporated into the daily schedule. In the acute stage a wet dressing with cold water is applied to promote blood flow, while a warm-water dressing may be advantageous in the chronic phase. Additional measures include physiotherapy, deep breathing exercises, yoga, acupuncture, electrotherapy, and local anaesthetics. In selected cases, orthopaedic supports may also contribute to alleviation of pain. Acute pain caused by fracture usually resolves within 10 weeks.

Chronic Phase: Short Term

Pain management may be
complicated by age-related
problems associated with
delay of metabolism and
excretion of medications.

The pain gradually eases as the fracture heals but can also merge into *chronic pain*, which is due to the development of a skeletal deformity after the fracture, as well as unbalanced and disproportionate strain on the muscles, and damage to the vertebral joints. Patients frequently complain of nocturnal pains (reminiscent of Sudeck-like pains) which respond to administration of nonsteroidal antiiflammatory agents. This chronic pain may be responsible for loss of sleep, irritability, fear, and depression, which in turn highlight the pain even more. Moreover, sensitivity to pain varies greatly between patients and each must be evaluated and treated individually. But the first priority in all patients is to break the spiral of pain and its consequences, and this is accomplished by physiotherapy and by analgetics, calcitonin (either subcutaneously or nasally), or bisphosphonates (intravenously). Other treatments to decrease pain in vertebral fractures include percutaneous injection of artificial cement into the vertebral body (see Chap. 11).

Chronic Phase: Long Term

Once the pain has become bearable, the patient must be mobilised and the muscles must be strengthened. This is best accomplished by *physiotherapy*, special exercises, and the ancillary measures noted above. Every patient should have an individualised program drawn up by the responsible physician in consultation with the physiotherapist. Swimming in particular, in warm or cold water, presents the ideal combination of relieving the vertebral column of weight while strengthening the muscles. As the pain lessens and the patient's condition improves, more sport-oriented measures are introduced. Active training to strengthen bones and muscles also contributes to reduction of chronic pain. Exercises should be performed regularly and be adapted to the patient's age. The program is developed and taught under specialist guidance to begin with and later should be continued by the patient in her/his home on a regular basis. A major aim is the stabilisation and strengthening of the muscles of the back – especially the lower thoracic and lumbar spine. Care must be taken to avoid exercises which carry an increased risk of vertebral fractures, especially those which flex the lumbar spine, increasing thoracic kyphosis and forward flexion.

Regular supervision of medication and physical activity is essential. Individual programmes must be designed and carried out.

Electric Potentials in Bone

It has long been recognised that weight bearing induces "stress lines" and thereby electric potentials in bone, which is very important for healing and for new bone formation. This phenomenon is called "piezolectricity" and it forms the basis for the theory that electrical charges constitute the impetus for bone resorption and formation. These electromagnetic fields in bone provide signals for neighboring bone cells to "remodel" the bone according to the immediate need or requirement. The "trajection lines" seen in X-ray pictures represent these stress lines exactly. The compact bone lies where the pressure points converge and the trabecular bone where they diverge. These characteristics have practical applications as they can be used to facilitate fracture healing as well as remodelling of newly-formed bone by means of a *"magnetic field therapy."* The physician in charge must check to find out for which indications this therapy has been approved. Examples are:

Electric field therapy is not yet widely used but has potential for the future.

▶ Delayed fracture healing
▶ Pseudoarthrosis
▶ Loosening of endoprosthesis

CHAPTER 12 Calcium and Vitamin D: The Skeleton's Best Friends

Calcium: A Lifelong Companion, From Infancy Onwards

Calcium is the most abundant mineral in the body and most of it – about 99% – is deposited in bone. There is no doubt that calcium is a fundamental player in prevention and treatment of osteoporosis. The calcium recommendation for adults is about 1,000 mg a day (higher for teenage girls, pregnant and lactating women, postmenopausal women who are not taking oestrogen, and men and women over age fifty). Today we ingest far less calcium than our ancestors did. In fact,

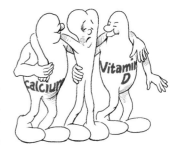

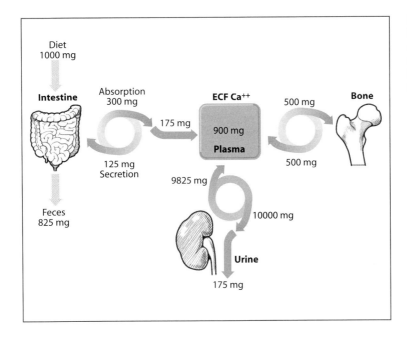

Fig. 12.1. Calcium metabolism in normal adult. Note distribution of calcium and excretion of large quantities in faeces and urine. *ECF*, extracellular fluid

Table 12.1. Amounts of elemental calcium in calcium salts used as supplements

Calcium salt	Calcium mg/ 1,000 mg calcium salt	% Calcium
Calcium carbonate	400	40.0
Calcium phosphate tribasic	388	38.8
Calcium lactate	184	18.4
Calcium gluconate	93	9.3
Calcium citrate	241	24.1

studies reveal that three-quarters of Americans are deficient in calcium, with an average of only 500–600 mg a day in their diet.

Numerous studies have shown that high calcium intake reduces postmenopausal bone loss and the risk of fractures, even in people who have already had fractures. Some evidence points to greater effectiveness in reducing bone loss perimenopausally than postmenopausally. Supplements of calcium (1,000–1,500 mg/day) and vitamin D alone have been shown to decrease the risk of fracture by 40%! Calcium supplementation at levels of 1,000 mg a day will suppress bone breakdown, probably by decreasing parathyroid hormone secretion. Increased calcium intake during adolescence helps to build up peak bone mass early in life, and the mineral stores laid down in the teens will definitely decrease the risk of osteoporosis in later years. While calcium by itself cannot treat or heal established osteoporosis, it appears to enhance the effectiveness of other treatments which inhibit resorption and/or promote formation.

> While calcium by itself won't treat established osteoporosis, it enhances the effectiveness of any treatment regimen.

The best way to get sufficient calcium is to eat foods rich in it. Getting enough calcium only with meals entails consumption of many other nutrients at the same time. Bottled mineral waters with high calcium content, low-fat dairy products, green leafy vegetables, and calcium-fortified juices will help to provide plenty of calcium. However, experience has shown that most patients do not get the required amount of calcium by nutrition alone. In this situation, *calcium supplements* are recommended and are available in tablet or powder, as well as in several other forms, each with its own advantages and disadvantages:

> It is a long journey from calcium in the mouth to calcium in the bones.

▶ Naturally derived calcium (dolomite, bonemeal, oyster shell): this type of supplement is inexpensive and easy to swallow, but it is harder to absorb and some sources may contain significant amounts of lead and other toxic minerals.

▶ Refined calcium carbonate is the least expensive form of calcium and has the highest percentage of elemental calcium, but it is poorly absorbed. It often causes constipation and because it is an antacid, in the long run it may lead to "rebound hyperacidity" and gastric irritation. It requires acid in order to dissolve. Taking calcium carbonate supplements together with vitamin C or with meals helps to some extent because that is when the stomach acid levels are highest.

▶ Chelated calcium is calcium bound to an organic acid, including citrate, citrate malate, lactate, gluconate, and others. Although chelated calcium is bulkier than calcium carbonate, it dissolves easily and therefore may be easier to absorb. In older patients, calcium citrate is preferred.

Very few patients cannot take calcium or only under medical supervision. Patients with hypercalcemia, nephrolithiasis, or renal insufficiency belong to this group. The following *points* may help in the choice of advantageous calcium supplements:

Calcium cannot work alone and needs special "helpers".

▶ Calcium is primarily absorbed in the small intestine, especially in the duodenum and proximal jejunum. Absorption of calcium is complete within 4 h. During periods of rapid skeletal growth, children reabsorb about 75% of ingested calcium, this value decreases to 30% in adults.

▶ Avoid taking more than 500 mg of calcium in one dose. Take one dose before bedtime to prevent bone loss at night. If more is needed, take several doses throughout the day.

▶ Calcium supplements should be taken with meals to boost their absorption, which is increased by lactose and proteins.

▶ Certain substances can hinder absorption of calcium: high-fibre and high-fat foods, zinc, iron, spinach, coffee, alcohol and antacids. Therefore, calcium should not be taken together with these.

▶ Patients should be advised to aim for a calcium – phosphorus ratio of 2:1. The easiest way to achieve this is to avoid excessive intake of cola drinks and foods with phosphorus additives.

▶ Calcium may interfere with certain drugs: thyroid medications, tetracyclin, anticonvulsants, and corticosteroids. Therefore, these should always be taken separately.

▶ There is no need to worry about kidney stone formation, when the right dosage and form of calcium are taken.

Mineral waters and calcium-fortified juices are good sources of minerals, but check the labels to find out what you get, as they vary widely in their calcium content.

▶ The amount of calcium in blood and urine should be checked regularly when supplements are taken.
▶ Calcium supplements can cause gas, abdominal distension, and constipation in some individuals. In this situation it is reasonable to switch to a different preparation.

Despite the linkage between calcium intake and bone mass, the incidence of osteoporosis is low in many areas, particularly in developing countries, where calcium intake is also low. There may be many possible explanations for this apparent paradox:

▶ Insufficient reports
▶ Lower life expectancies
▶ Nondietary factors (genetic differences, exercise patterns, exposure to sunlight)
▶ Dietary factors (consumption of soy and other natural products)

Vitamin D: Don't Rely on Sunshine, Take Supplements

In addition to its regulation of calcium, vitamin D has many other beneficial effects – in all age groups.

Vitamin D is one of the most important regulators of calcium, having the following actions which effect the skeleton:

▶ Promotes absorption of calcium from the gut into the blood-stream
▶ Decreases the excretion of calcium in the kidney
▶ Promotes the recruitment, maturation, and action of bone cells
▶ Promotes the incorporation of calcium into bone (mineralisation)
   Additional beneficial *actions of vitamin D* are:
▶ Increase of muscle mass and strength
▶ Improvement of coordination
▶ Lower risk of falling
▶ Decrease of systolic blood pressure
▶ Lower risk of breast and colon cancer
▶ Anti-inflammatory action

Vitamin D is measured in international units (IU). The recommended daily intake of vitamin D is 200–400 IU, but this is a maintenance amount and is not enough for therapeutic effects, for which 400–1,000 IU are considered to be effective. Most people deficient in vitamin D readily agree to take supplements and not rely on dietary intake.

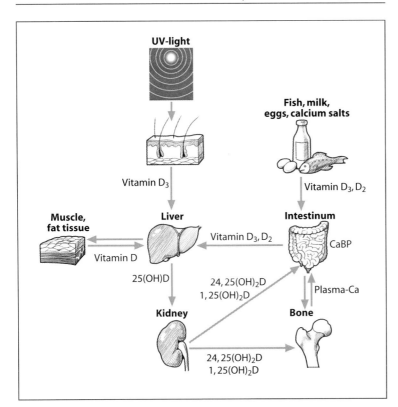

Fig. 12.2. Pathways of vitamin D metabolism. *CaBP*, calcium binding protein

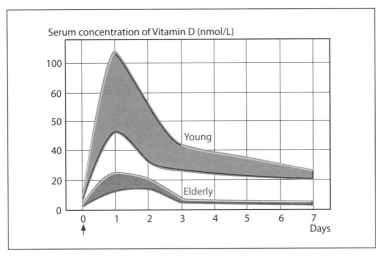

Fig. 12.3. Decreasing ability of the skin to produce vitamin D in response to exposure to sunlight. (Modified from Holick et al. [Lancet 1989, 4:1104–1105])

Rickets is a childhood disease resulting from vitamin D deficiency. In adults, the resulting disease is called *osteomalacia*. A relative vitamin D deficiency often occurs in older age groups and in people with disorders of the gastrointestinal tract. The following factors contribute to a *calcium/vitamin D deficiency in older people*:

▶ Inadequate consumption of calcium-rich foods
▶ Reduced absorption capacity of the intestinal mucosa
▶ Reduced exposure to sunlight, and therefore
▶ Reduced synthesis of vitamin D in the skin
▶ Reduced metabolism of vitamin D to its active form

The conclusion to be drawn from this survey of calcium and vitamin D metabolism: both must be taken regularly by everybody in the right quantity – 1,000 mg calcium plus 1,000 IU vitamin D

As a consequence of these factors, most elderly patients have some degree of secondary hyperparathyroidism with increased bone resorption. Vitamin D supplements bring about a decrease of the serum PTH concentration, a decrease of bone turnover, and an increase of bone mineral density. Vitamin D and calcium supplements could decrease the incidence of hip and other peripheral fractures in nursing home residents. Therefore, prescription of 1,000 mg calcium and 1,000 IU vitamin D daily for prevention of involutional or age-related osteoporosis is indicated and highly recommended. Alternatively, 150,000 IU i.m. every 6 months can be prescribed if there are difficulties in compliance or to avoid them.

Vitamin D is especially important in *childhood* during growth. Growing children need vitamin D for:

▶ Increased absorption of calcium from food
▶ Recruitment, maturation, and activation of bone-forming cells
▶ Mineralisation and hardening of new bone

An adequate supply of vitamin D (recommended dose of 1,000 IU daily) is therefore extremely important for normal development of the skeleton.

Vitamin D is fat-soluble and therefore the body can store it. Supplemental vitamin D seems to enhance the benefit from calcium.

Vitamin D belongs to the group of fat-soluble vitamins such as Vitamin A, E, and K and therefore can be stored in the body for long periods. Patients suffering from conditions which reduce absorption of fat usually also have deficiencies of these vitamins. Such patients are best treated by one of the many multivitamin preparations available. The conclusion which must be drawn from this brief review of calcium and vitamin D is that in the framework of osteoporosis prevention and therapy everybody must receive 1,000 mg calcium and 1,000 IU vitamin D either in food or in supplements every day throughout the year. In the elderly with poor nutritional status there may be some benefit from protein and multivitamin supplementation.

Could Too Much Calcium and Vitamin D Be Harmful?

Recently *upper limits* for both calcium and vitamin D have been recommended for children of one year and older: calcium =2,500 mg/day and vitamin D = 2,000 IU (50 µg)/day. When consumed in very high quantities, both calcium and vitamin D can cause health risks. High calcium intake may decrease absorption of other minerals such as iron and zinc. The risk of kidney stones, however, is a complex issue because there are many causes of renal stones. In general, adequate dietary calcium does not increase the risk of calcium oxalate stones by binding to oxalate in the intestine. The potential risk of excessive vitamin D intake includes damage to the central nervous system, which in turn can result in depression, nausea, and anorexia. With increasing availability of supplements and fortified foods, it will be important to monitor intakes of these substances. The dose of calcium supplement should be adjusted based on dietary intakes.

Could "too much of a good thing" damage health? Yes, so check quantities and don't overdo it, especially as vitamin D is fat-soluble and is stored in the body.

Is Activated Vitamin D Better Than the Native Form?

Vitamin D metabolism is inhibited in patients with chronic renal and hepatic disorders, so that the activated form of vitamin D is required for these patients, in whom they stabilise and may even increase bone mass. Activated vitamin D metabolites are physiological and therefore nontoxic substances, but they are metabolically highly active so that levels of calcium in blood and urine must be checked regularly to exclude hypo- or hypercalcemia and/or hypercalciuria with stone formation. No more than 500 mg calcium per day can be given to these patients. Recommended dosages are:

Alfacalcidol   0.5–1.0 µg/day orally
Calcitriol   0.5 µg/day orally

Other Vitamins of Clinical Relevance

Vitamin K is also important in normal bone formation. A higher vitamin K intake helps prevent hip fractures. Vitamin K appears to be essential for conversion of osteocalcin to its active form in bone. There are three major forms of vitamin K:

▶ K1 (phylloquinone) is the natural form found in plants, especially in leafy, dark-green vegetables
▶ K2 (menaquinone) is produced by bacteria in the gut
▶ K3 (menadione) is a synthetic form

The recommended dose for vitamin K is 100–300 IU daily. Vitamin K is particularly important for management of bone loss in patients with hepatic cirrhosis.

Vitamin A in excess may be detrimental to bone, and intakes of more than 1,500 µg RE/d are related to a twofold increased risk of hip fracture in some studies.

Further nutritional supplements for healthy bones are *magnesium* and four essential *trace elements*: boron, silicon, zinc, and copper. Magnesium plays several roles in the metabolism of vitamin D and in the regulation of parathyroid hormone. Finally, osseous alkaline phosphatase is activated by magnesium. Some studies have found that higher magnesium intakes are associated with higher BMD in the elderly. However, magnesium supplementation is only recommended in magnesium-depleted individuals. The recommended daily dose of magnesium is 200–500 mg.

Vitamin K is going to be the "new" bone-building vitamin.

Vitamins A, D, E and K are fat-soluble and so can be stored by the body. That means that you can give a supplement with a higher dose once a month.

CHAPTER 13

**Hormones for Replacement:
A Matter of Re-Evaluation**

Hormone Replacement Therapy (HRT) for Women: Now Recommended Only for Symptoms and for Short Periods Only

Decrease in oestrogen production starts well before menopause and initiates a continuous loss of bone. After menopause, in the absence of therapy 1%–4% of bone mass may be lost annually. In general, the indications for HRT were:

► Relief of postmenopausal symptoms and signs attributable to oestrogen deficiency
► Reduction of risk of diseases associated with oestrogen deficiency (osteoporosis and cardio/cerebrovascular disorders)
► HRT was thought to delay cognitive decline, but this has not been substantiated

Long-term use (5–10 years) of oestrogen results in reduction of fractures of the hip, vertebrae, and arm by about 50%. The greatest effect is seen in the vertebral column: within 2 years of HRT increases of up to 10% in bone density of the lumbar vertebrae, and up to 4% in the femoral neck have been reported. The effect of HRT is more pronounced in skeletal sites with mainly trabecular bone. When HRT is stopped, bone loss immediately resumes at the usual postmenopausal rate.

Although oestrogen is considered to be the gold standard for osteoporosis prevention, not all patients experience an increase in bone mass. Because of this, the National Osteoporosis Foundation recommends BMD-testing for all women on long-term hormone replacement to assure that the patient has responded to this treatment. In patients who have not responded adequately to oestrogen therapy or in

The loss of oestrogen at menopause triggers a period of rapid bone loss of about 5 years. During this time, the skeleton is relatively resistant to intervention with calcium alone. By 5–8 years after the menopause, the rate of bone loss declines from an average of 3% to about 1% per year.

those found to have very low bone mass, a combination of HRT and alendronate has shown additive benefits on bone and should be considered.

Every woman who reaches menopause is therefore confronted with the far-reaching decision as to whether or not to begin HRT. Some authors use the term HRT for combined oestrogen-progesterone, and ERT when only oestrogen is used. It is advisable to reach a decision concerning HRT only after consultation with the patient and with a gynaecologist. However, today the indications are far more limited and the operative principles are:

▶ Who gets HRT? – as few women as possible
▶ How much HRT? – as little as possible
▶ For how long? – as short as possible

The *mechanisms of action* of oestrogen on bone are complex and include:

▶ Inhibition of osteoclast activity
▶ Stimulation of collagen synthesis by osteoblasts
▶ Promotion of gastrointestinal absorption of calcium
▶ Stimulation of calcitonin secretion
▶ Modulation of parathyroid hormone secretion
▶ Improvement of central nervous functions and therefore decrease of tendency to fall
▶ Increased blood flow through the bone

HRT: for symptoms only!   The data from the oestrogen/progesterone arm of the *Women's Health Initiative Study (2003)* has affected perceptions on the effects of HRT and its role in management. The study has confirmed that HRT reduces the risk of vertebral, nonvertebral, and hip fractures. This is a major advance in the evidence base concerning the effect of HRT on bone but at the same time, cardiovascular and breast cancer data from the trial have had a negative effect on perceptions. As a result, a majority of women who use HRT will limit their use to the decade following menopause. Women at high risk of osteoporosis who wish to minimise postmenopausal bone loss, yet who do not wish to continue HRT over a long time, should consider the option of transferring to raloxifene or a nitrogen-containing bisphosphonate.

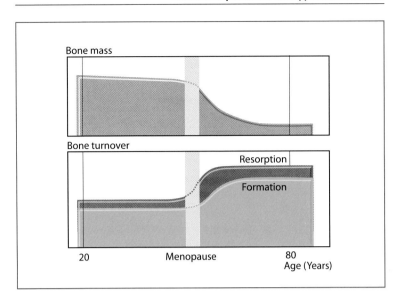

Fig. 13.1. Changes in bone mass, resorption, and formation before and at menopause, without therapy

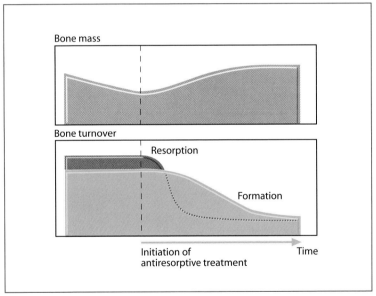

Fig. 13.2. Preservation and/or increase in bone mass, decrease in bone turnover at and after menopause under the influence of bisphosphonate therapy

Which Oestrogens and Progestins, and How to Take Them?

The main groups of oestrogen preparations given orally or transdermally are:

▶ Synthetic oestrogen analogues with a steroid skeleton
▶ Nonhuman oestrogen, produced from an equine source (conjugated equine oestrogens)
▶ Native human oestrogens or compounds that are transformed to native oestrogens in the body.

Effective daily doses of commonly used oestrogens are:

Oestradiol	Orally	2 mg
	Patch	50 µg
	Gel	1 mg
Conjugated equine oestrogens	0.625 mg	
Oestradiol valerate	2 mg	

For women with an intact uterus, oestrogen should be combined with *progestin* to prevent the risk of endometrial hyperplasia and cancer. Cyclic treatment is recommended for women immediately after menopause, while continuous daily intake is suitable for older women when regular uterine bleeding is undesirable. Most clinical experience has been gained with the use of medroxyprogesterone acetate, norethisterone acetate and levonorgestrel.

Tibolone is a synthetic analogue of gonadal steroids with combined oestrogenic, progestogenic, and androgenic properties. The endometrium is unaffected and combination with progestin is not necessary. At a dose of 2.5 mg daily it reduces bone turnover by 30%–50% and so increases bone mass by 2%–5% during the first 2 years. This effect on bone is similar to that of conventional HRT. The effect on fracture risk remains to be determined.

Which Women to Treat?

Early treatment is warranted for the following indications:

▶ Premature and surgically induced menopause, especially below the age of 40

► Osteopenic women (T-score <1 SD)
► Loss of bone density in excess of 1% per year (DEXA)
► Women at high risk because of life style or other factors

How Long to Treat?

Every patient must decide for herself how long to continue to take HRT. For effective prevention and management of osteoporosis a period of 5–15 years is recommended, possibly even for life. The longer the therapy, the longer the bone is protected. HRT can be started even at 75 years of age, but must be continued and taken regularly, to avoid undesirable side effects. As soon as HRT is discontinued, bone resorption begins again, so that the bone density returns to its starting value 3–4 years after cessation of therapy. Research on the discontinuation of HRT has demonstrated that the rate of loss of bone mass is similar to the rate of loss at menopause.

Research has shown that up to 25-30% of oestrogen prescriptions are never filled and about 50% of patients who begin HRT discontinue treatment within 6 months.

The general compliance with HRT is low and women often reject HRT:

► Only 15% of women who would benefit from HRT actually take it.
► Only 70%–50% of the various oestrogen preparations prescribed are actually taken.
► Only 20% of women who embarked on therapy with oestrogen take it for more than 5 years.

Compliance can be increased by better information and support under treatment, which should be only for symptoms and only for short periods. For many women, life style changes, increased physical activity, proper nutrition and supplements would prevent osteoporosis and obviate the need for hormones.

How to Monitor HRT?

Oestrogen replacement therapy, with or without progestin, needs to be monitored annually for efficacy and safety:

► *Efficacy:* DEXA, Alkaline phosphatase, and Crosslaps in the serum, selectively oestradiol and sex hormone-binding globulin (SHBG)

▶ *Safety*: Annual breast examination and mammogram, vaginal ultrasound

Some patients may not respond to oral oestrogens because of gastrointestinal side effects, malabsorption or enterohepatic binding of oestrogen. Alternative routes of administration include oestrogen patches or gel.

What Are the Risks and Adverse Events of HRT?

Patients can be discouraged taking HRT by the inconvenience of periodic bleeding, distressing mood swings, fear of breast or uterine cancer and fear of stroke, hypertension and thrombosis.

Over the past few years many studies have been designed, carried out, and published on the risk and benefits of HRT, especially long-term. HRT has been taken for many years by millions of women after cessation of the menses. Results of recent controlled trials do not show a protective effect of HRT on reducing risk of coronary artery disease, but there was a decreased risk of colorectal cancer and osteoporotic fractures. Most importantly however, there was an increased risk of heart disease, stroke, invasive breast cancer and venous thromboembolism. The findings of these extensive, controlled trials have seriously undermined the indications for long-term HRT, which should no longer be prescribed. "Better safe than sorry" as the proverb has it!

Despite some 50 observational studies, there is still no complete consensus on breast cancer risk with HRT. Most experts agree that oestrogen may be a promoter rather than a cause of breast cancer. The risk of breast cancer for ERT-treated women appears to be time- and dose-dependent and increases by 25%–70% after 10–15 years of ERT. In the *HERS study*, the use of oestrogen in women with serious cardiovascular disease did not result in a protection against myocardial infarction. A further large prospective study (*Woman's Health Initiative*) designed to answer many questions related to oestrogen replacement included more than 27,000 older, generally healthy postmenopausal women. The oestrogen-plus-progesterin segment was stopped when results showed that hormone therapy caused small increases in the risk of coronary events, stroke, pulmonary embolism, and breast cancer. There were also some small decreases in the risks of hip fracture and colon cancer, but the overall harm outweighed these benefits. There was also clear evidence that hormone therapy does not result in better quality of life among older women without menopausal symptoms, and does not improve cognition, depression, or sexual function.

Women with vasomotor symptoms must weigh the risks associated with treatment against the benefits of symptom relief. They require treatment for a much shorter duration than 5 years, and therefore the risk will be smaller. Given the availability of other effective drugs, the use of hormone therapy for the prevention or treatment of osteoporosis is not appropriate for most women. Obviously, the indications for HRT have changed as have the variety of choices available and alternative therapies.

What Are the Main Contraindications?

▶ Vaginal bleeding of unknown origin
▶ Thrombotic tendency and pulmonary emboli
   in the patient's history
▶ Family history of breast cancer
▶ Hypertension
▶ Acute or chronic hepatic disorders
▶ Hypertriglyceridemia
▶ Malignant melanoma

There are individual contraindications to HRT and each patient must be checked before even short-term HRT is prescribed.

Natural Oestrogens: How Effective Are They?

There is much interest among postmenopausal women in "natural" alternatives to oestrogen. Phyto-oestrogens, also known as plant oestrogens, are nonsteroidal molecules (isoflavones, lignans, coumestans, stilbenes, and resorcyclic lactones) and occur naturally in plants and vegetables, for example, in soy products, some types of peas and beans, as well as in tea, milk, and beer. These plants contain three main classes of phyto-oestrogens: isoflavones, lignans, and coumestans, which resemble oestrogen chemically and are converted in the body into very weak forms of oestrogen. These molecules do not share the common chemical structure with oestrogens, but they have two structural features that resemble oestrogens:

▶ An aromatic A ring with an hydroxyl group, and
▶ A second hydroxyl group in the same plane of the A ring.

Fig. 13.3. Similar action of oestrogens and phyto-oestrogens in stimulating osteoblasts to produce proteins which constitute bone matrix. *ER*, estrogen receptor; *MAPK*, mitogen-activated protein kinase. (Modified from Migliaccio and Anderson [A95])

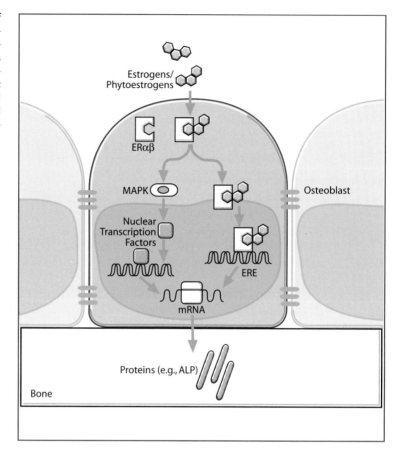

Recent trials have failed to establish a beneficial effect of phyto-oestrogens on bone density.

These similarities allow the molecules to bind to the oestrogen receptors (ER) and thereby lead to biological activity (nuclear DNA-stimulated protein synthesis).

Though these plant oestrogens are a thousand times weaker than animal oestrogens, they do exercise a positive effect on the vegetative manifestations of the menopause and they also have positive effects on bone building. Isoflavones are found principally in legumes and soybean products. In terms of dietary sources, most soy products contain about 2 mg/g of isoflavones, and the upper limit of isoflavone intake should be approximately 50 mg/day from diet and supplements. Lignans are found in fruits, vegetables and beer, and coumestans in

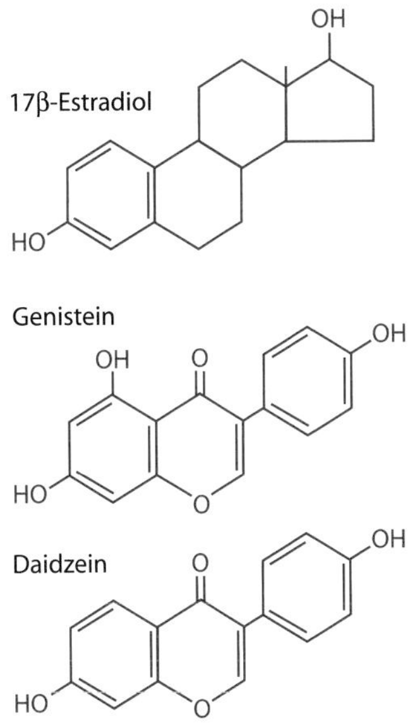

Fig. 13.4. Structures of the 17β-oestradiol and the two main natural oestrogens found in soy. (Genistein and Daidzein)

bean sprouts and fodder crops. Two small studies have demonstrated that they significantly reduced the fracture risk. An additional advantage is that, presumably, they have no tumour-promoting activity. The recommended dose of ipriflavone is 600 mg daily, taken in two or three separate doses. Though these results are promising, larger studies are necessary to demonstrate the value of phyto-oestrogens in osteoporosis. Phyto-oestrogens have the potential of significant biological effects, although the spectrum of these effects may be quite different from that of oestrogen or SERMs. However, cell and animal studies have shown that this effect is mediated, at least in part, via the classical oestrogen receptor mechanism, presumably via the osteoblasts. Stimulation of both cell proliferation and alkaline phosphatase, a marker of osteoblastic cell differentiation, suggests that genistein may enhance bone formation activities. Genistein also inhibits the synthesis and secretion of interleukin-6, which further indicates that this substance may decrease osteoclast differentiation and function through an osteoblast-mediated effect, as already suggested for E2.

Soy is the queen of plant proteins and phyto-oestrogens.

The safety of pharmacological doses of phytooestrogens is unknown.

Recommendations for the medical community and the general public concerning the use of soy and other isoflavone supplements to help postmenopausal women with low BMD must await further randomized clinical trials to satisfy objectively the needs for evidence-based medicine. One must also keep in mind that herbal products are not regulated by the FDA, which means that the purity, safety, and effectiveness of the herb is not necessarily assured and the amount of active drug per milligram dose may vary with different manufacturers. There may also be the possibility of contamination with other compounds, when collected, distilled, and manufactured in capsules. Furthermore, the metabolism of the active drugs and consequently their action appear to be highly influenced by other factors of the diet, intestinal function, intestinal bacteria, and individual variations. However, standardized plant extracts as substitutes for HRT are now available and results of trials are awaited.

Dehydroepiandrosterone (DHEA): Is It Useful for Prevention of Bone Loss?

DHEA – a rising star for osteoporosis prevention?

This substance has gained a great deal of attention from the media and the public and many people now take DHEA to prevent or reverse various age-related changes. DHEA is one of the major circulating adrenal androgens. Serum DHEA levels peak by the second decade of life and then steadily decline by about 10 % per decade. The regulatory role of DHEA in bone metabolism has been evaluated in several studies, indicating that adrenal androgens may prevent bone loss induced by oestrogen deficiency. When using pharmacological doses of DHEA, variable effects on blood lipids and body composition have been reported, but none of these studies investigated the effects on bones. Consequently, DHEA supplements should be deferred until the results of ongoing studies with this hormone are published.

Testosterone: Good for Bones and Well-being in Men

Secondary osteoporosis should always be suspected if a decrease in bone density occurs in a young male. Possibilities are hypogonadism or Klinefelter syndrome, for which the therapy of choice is early institution of *testosterone replacement therapy*. Hypogonadism in the male is associated with low values of calcitriol and decreased intestinal absorption of calcium. Under therapy with testosterone, gains in BMD correlated better with serum oestrogen levels than with testosterone, indicating that conversion of testosterone to oestrogen may be an important factor. Treatment may also increase muscle mass and improve well-being. The use of testosterone therapy should be limited to men with low levels of free testosterone who have no contraindications such as prostatic hypertrophy or prostate cancer). Safety of treatment should be monitored by blood count, and of levels of glucose and prostate-specific antigen (PSA). Recommendations for testosterone replacement in patients with low serum levels are intramuscular injections 100–250 mg every 3–4 weeks or testosterone gel 5 mg daily.

> The use of testosterone therapy should be limited to men with low levels of free testosterone who have no contraindications to the use of this hormone.

Anabolic Steroids: Strong Muscles for Healthy Bones

The efficacy of these drugs in osteoporosis has long been recognised and is due to their effect on the muscles, although a direct action on bone-forming cells has also been described. These drugs are indicated in the elderly when there is muscular weakness or even cachexia. Anabolic steroid therapy in the elderly has a significant anabolic effect on bone in addition to its anticatabolic effect. Treatment should be restricted to 3 years, and the well-known side effects (virilisation in women) and hepatic damage must be taken into consideration. Moreover, men may experience a reduction in sexual function. In addition, cancer of the prostate must be ruled out before therapy is started, because it could be stimulated by anabolics. *Nandrolone* decanoate is the most utilised preparation and is injected i.m. in a dose of 50 mg every 4 weeks. This drug can also be used as adjuvant treatment in elderly women as well as in male patients with osteoporosis.

> The decline in bone mass is roughly parallel with a decline in muscle mass and strength.

CHAPTER 14 Bisphosphonates: The Success Story in Osteoporosis

Bisphosphonates: little short of a wonder drug in osteology!

A new era in the treatment of disorders of bone began about 30 years ago with the introduction of bisphosphonates into clinical practice. Bisphosphonates are deposited on the surface of the bone and inhibit osteoclasts and thus resorption of bone. Consequently, these drugs have long been given to patients with Morbus Paget, hypercalcemia, and osseous metastases. Bisphosphonates not only inhibit resorption of bone, they also inhibit growth of metastases in the bone and in the bone marrow.

Bisphosphonates inhibit resorption in osteoporosis and – at least the aminobisphosphonates – have no adverse effects on bone formation and therefore lead to a long-lasting (periods of years) positive bone balance. Bisphosphonates have been successfully used for prevention and therapy in all forms of osteoporosis. Compact and spongy bone show equal increases in bone density. Moreover, the long-term incorporation of bisphosphonates into the bones has no detectable deleterious influence on bone quality and strength. The concept of "frozen bone" under bisphosphonate therapy is simply false; a basic level of remodelling is consistently maintained even under bisphosphonate therapy. Disturbances of mineralisation have not been observed with the new bisphosphonates currently in use.

Bisphosphonates have now been successfully used for prevention and therapy of osteoporosis in both sexes, at all ages, in all conditions and in all forms of osteoporosis immaterial of the cause.

The nitrogen-containing bisphosphonates are today the most effective medications available for treatment of all forms of osteoporosis in both men and women, in young and old, in congenital and acquired, in primary and secondary, in high and low turnover, and in pre-, peri-, and postmenopausal osteoporoses. Bisphosphonates have also been given to children – even very young ones – but this should be done in recognised paediatric centres under strictly controlled indications and conditions.

A Brief Survey of Bisphosphonates

These are synthetic compounds, analogues of pyrophosphate in which the oxygen atom of the central P-O-P bond has been replaced by carbon, resulting in a P-C-P group. This exchange has made the bisphosphonates resistant to enzymatic hydrolysis. In addition, different bisphosphonates can be synthesised by substitution of both hydrogen atoms on the carbon atom, and these bisphosphonates differ in their biological properties, their activities, their pharmacodynamics, and their toxicity. There are two side chains:

Bisphosphonates rapidly deposit on the bone surface, explaining why practically only bone is affected.

▶ One binds to bone mineral
▶ One determines class and potency (nitrogen molecule)

The dynamics of these new bisphosphonates manifest themselves in their potency – they are 20,000 times more potent than etidronate, the first generation bisphosphonate. Bisphosphonates have a high affinity for certain structures on the surface of bone. Most of the bisphosphonate absorbed in the gastrointestinal tract is deposited on bone within hours especially in resorption bays (Howship's lacunae) or in the acid environment under the osteoclasts. This causes a most effective inhibition of osteoclasts and of resorption, as well as reactivation of

Table 14.1. List of available bisphosphonates according to side chains and relative potency

Substance	Trade name	R1	R2	Relative potency
Etidronate	Didronel	–OH	–CH$_3$	1×
Clodronate	Ostac, Bonefos	–Cl	–Cl	10×
Pamidronate	Aredia	–OH	–CH$_2$–CH$_2$–NH$_2$	100×
Alendronate	Fosamax	–OH	–CH$_2$–CH$_2$–CH$_2$–NH$_2$	1,000×
Risedronate	Actonel	–OH	–CH$_2$– (ring)	5,000×
Ibandronate	Bondronat	–OH	–CH$_2$–CH$_2$–NH$_2$–CH$_3$ C$_5$H$_{11}$	10,000×
Zoledronate	Zometa	–OH	–CH$_2$–N (ring)	20,000×

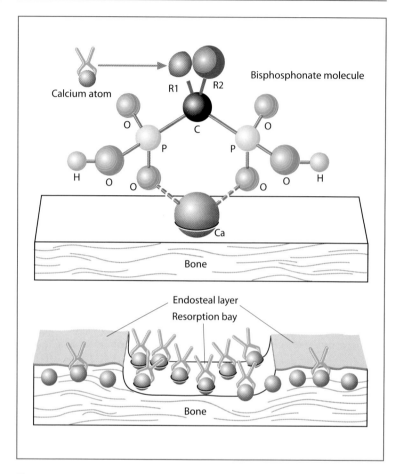

Fig. 14.1. Molecular structure of bisphosphonates. Note structural resemblance to tongs. Deposition of bisphosphonates on osseous surface: subsequently bisphosphonates are phagocytosed by osteoclasts or incorporated into bone

Fig. 14.2. Cellular and biochemical mechanisms of action of bisphosphonates. ▶ Active osteoclast: bisphosphonate molecules in fluid interphase between osteoclast and bone. Phagocytosed bisphosphonates inhibit osteoclastic enzymes, shown by detraction of ruffled membrane, and induce apoptosis

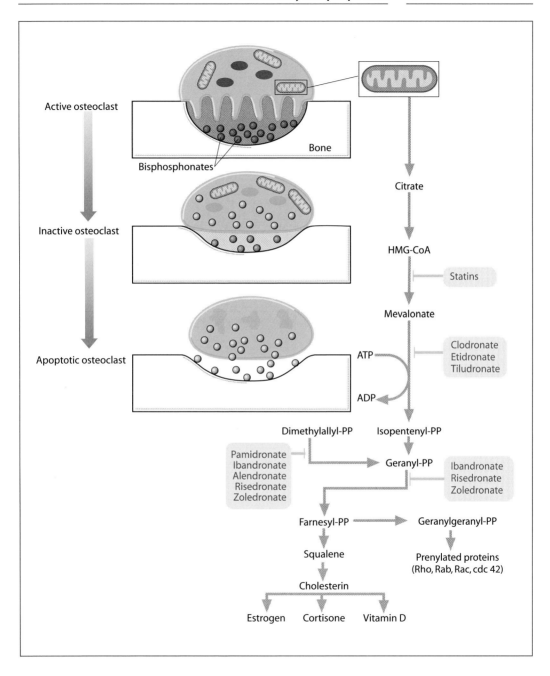

The skeletal retention of bisphosphonates is very long, sometimes lifelong.

the suppressed osteoblasts and thereby an overall positive "bone balance" and increase in bone mass. The bisphosphonates deposited on the surface are later (weeks or months) built into the bone and may remain there for many years, until eventually they may reach the surface again in a remodelling cycle. However, due to their extremely low concentrations, these bisphosphonates remain inactive, even when "recycled," that is, when the bone on which they are deposited undergoes remodelling again.

The *mechanism of action* is not yet completely understood, but some aspects have been elucidated:

► Incorporation of bisphosphonates into hydroxyapatite crystals and into the bone matrix leads to decreased solubility of the bone substance and disturbances of mineralisation – physical-chemical effect

► Reduction in recruitment and in fusion of osteoclast precursors – direct influence on the monocyte-macrophage system

► Inhibition of osteoclast activity by means of inhibition of the proton-ATPases – a direct toxic effect

► Inhibition of enzymes of mevalonic acid metabolism – by the aminobisphosphonates

► Shortening of osteoclastic survival by induction of apoptosis, probably associated with a lengthening of osteoblastic survival (alterations in the periods of the phases of the remodelling cycles)

► Indirect inhibition of osteoclastic resorption by way of factors produced by osteoblasts – interference with "coupling" in the osteoblast-osteoclast cycle

► Increased synthesis of collagen type I by osteoblasts

► Inhibition of production of prostaglandin E2, of proteolytic enzymes, of interleukin 1 and 6, and many other cytokines

► Inhibition of adherence of osteoclasts and tumour cells to the surface of bone

► Effect on afferent nerve fibres in bone with inhibition of release of neuropeptides and neuromodulators at the nerve ends

From a laboratory point of view, inhibition of osteoclastic resorption results in decreased excretion of the breakdown products of collagen in the urine and a reduction in the level of calcium in the blood in patients with hypercalcemia. In the long term, inhibition of resorption results in a positive calcium balance with a continuous increase in

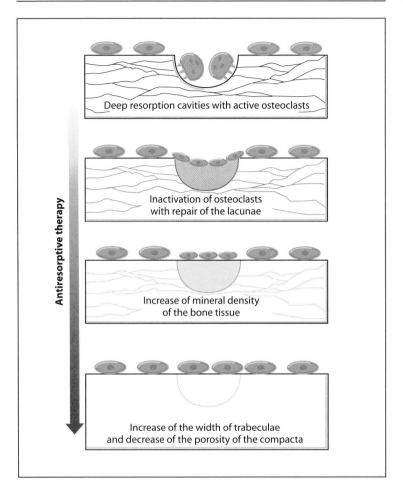

Fig. 14.3. Schematic illustration of sequence of effects of bisphosphonate therapy

bone mass, especially in trabecular bone because of its large surface area. Moreover, the increase in bone mass is accompanied by an increase in mechanical resistance of the bone. Bisphosphonates and other antiresorptive agents improve *bone strength* by various effects:

▶ They reduce the size of the remodelling space and repair the resorption cavities caused by increased osteoclastic activity.
▶ They maintain the trabecular architecture, especially the horizontal trabeculae.

▶ They decrease cortical porosity.
▶ They increase mineralisation density by a prolongation of the bone formation period.
▶ They maintain osteocytic viability. Indeed, recent studies indicate that osteocytes act as mechanosensors and thereby participate in regulation of bone remodelling. There is also evidence that oestrogen, bisphosphonates, and raloxifene all prevent osteocytic apoptosis.

Modern bisphosphonates do not interface with mineralisation, therefore there is no osteomalacia even after long-term use.

The osteomalacia (disturbance of mineralisation) observed after long-term use of the first generation of bisphosphonates has not occurred with the latest aminobisphosphonates (i. e., those with an aminogroup in one of the side chains) even after 8 years of therapy. Changes in lamellar structure of the trabeculae were also not observed. It has recently been reported that in dogs given six times the therapeutic dose of alendronate or risedronate, both of which substantially decrease bone turnover, there was an increase in histological microcracks. However, there was a greater increase in bone strength in the alendronate and in the risedronate groups than in controls. To summarise, in humans none of the currently used aminobisphosphonates were found to have any deleterious effects on bone quality, estimated by preclinical mechanical testing and clinical fracture risk.

In the future, bisphosphonates will also be used for prevention of skeletal metastases.

The most recent investigations have shown an antiproliferative effect of bisphosphonates on growth of tumour cells. The inhibition of osteoclasts results in a reduction in the production of IL6 and in the release of growth factors from the bone matrix. Evidence is also accumulating that bisphosphonates have a negative influence on osseous and probably also on visceral metastases possibly by way of interactions with adhesion molecules on the tumour cells, and/or by forming a film on the surface of the bone.

Pharmacokinetics

As mentioned above, the P-C-P bond is completely resistant to enzymatic hydrolysis. Consequently, the currently used bisphosphonates are absorbed unchanged, deposited on bone, and eventually excreted. They are not metabolised in the body, and interactions with other medications do not occur. Intestinal absorption is minimal – somewhere between 1% and 10%, and for the latest bisphosphonates probably less than 1%. Absorption may be further reduced if bisphosphonates are taken with food or drink, especially with bivalent salts such as calcium and magnesium. Consequently it is essential to ingest the bisphosphonates on an empty stomach and only with water. The manufacturers recommend taking alendronate and risedronate with a full glass of tap water on an empty stomach half an hour before breakfast. The patient must remain in an upright position to ensure absorption and to avoid adverse reactions. The tablet should not be regurgitated together with gastric juices and remain in the oesophagus because that could damage the mucus membrane. If a patient has difficulties in swallowing or there is a pre-existing reflux oesophagitis, an alternative therapy should be chosen. Of the absorbed bisphosphonate, 20%–50% adheres to the active bone surface; the rest is excreted in the urine or the faeces during the day.

In contrast to its short stay in the peripheral blood (half-life of 1–15 h) the *half-life of bisphosphonates in the skeleton* is much longer – a matter of years, as is the case for other substances with a high affinity for bones such as tetracyclin. Individual bisphosphonates may have different interactions with bone that result in differences in their pharmacological behaviour. For example, risedronate has lower kinetic binding affinity for the mineral substrates on bone surface than alendronate does. These differences may contribute to the apparent shorter terminal half-life of risedronate and to faster clinical on- and off-responses seen with risedronate compared to alendronate. Preliminary results suggest that ibandronate and zoledronate have higher kinetic binding affinities than alendronate and risedronate.

Bisphosphonates have a short half-life in the circulation, but a very long half-life in the bones.

Renal clearance of bisphosphonates is accomplished by active tubular excretion. The dose and half-life of the bisphosphonate given to patients with renal insufficiency and on haemodialysis must be carefully calculated for each individual patient.

Toxicity and Contraindications

Bisphosphonates are very well tolerated when taken as prescribed. Side effects and adverse reactions are few and rarely severe:

▶ *Gastrointestinal complaints* reported in 2%–10% of the patients include nausea, vomiting, stomach aches, and diarrhoea. However, in large placebo-controlled studies these were reported equally in both groups. Inflammation and ulceration of the oesophagus, occasionally reported, can easily be avoided by strict adherence to the directions for taking the medication. These lesions of the mucus membrane occur in two stages. Regurgitation of gastric acid dam-

Bisphosphonates are poorly absorbed, especially in the presence of food and calcium.

ages the oesophageal epithelium. Aminobisphosphonates diffuse into the adjoining epithelial cells and inhibit synthesis of cholesterin (inhibition of the mevalonic acid pathway), which in turn prevents cholesterin-dependent repair of the damaged mucosal cells. Bed-ridden patients or patients with reflux oesophagitis should not be given oral aminobisphosphonates, or at best only under the strictest medical supervision.

▶ *Acute phase reaction*: This can occur within 24 h of the first intravenous infusion of an aminobisphosphonate. The reaction consists of a rise in temperature, joint and bone pains, myalgias, increase of IL6 and C reactive proteins, and changes in lymphocyte counts.

▶ Very rarely, an infusion or oral treatment must be stopped because of the outbreak of a *skin allergy* or photosensibility.

▶ Very rarely, *ocular reactions* have been observed (1/1,000 patients). Uveitis scleritis and episcleritis have been observed after pamidronate. With cessation of the infusion and administration of glucocorticoids, the ocular inflammation improved rapidly.

▶ About 3 % of patients who receive infusions of bisphosphonates experience *moderate hypocalcemia and hypomagnesemia*, which, however, do not require any medical treatment. Aminobisphosphonates should not be given together with aminoglycosides since both medications reduce the calcium level in the blood, which may last for considerable periods of time. We have not observed any clinically significant hypocalcemia as a consequence of infusion of bisphosphonates.

Bisphosphonates should not be infused rapidly in large quantities, causing formation of insoluble aggregates which may impair renal function.

▶ *Renal function* should be checked before intravenous infusion of bisphosphonates. At high dosages, kidney pain may occur as well as mild, clinically nonsignificant albuminuria.

Nitrogen-containing bisphosphonates can be taken without risk by patients with fractures. They do not inhibit or delay repair!

▶ No human data suggest that the administration of modern bisphosphonates, at least in doses used for osteoporosis, interfere clinically with *fracture repair*. The amount of the callus was either not changed or was increased, but never decreased. The slowing of callus turnover was accompanied paradoxically by a higher mechanical strength.

▶ *Acute and chronic toxicity studies* using oral alendronate in female animals showed no evidence of mutagenicity, including those most relevant to human carcinogenic potential. Carcinogenicity studies in rats and mice at maximum tolerated doses showed no increase in tumour incidence associated with alendronate treatment. There was also no effect on fertility or reproductive performance in male or female rats.

Contraindications. Bisphosphonates should be avoided during pregnancy and breast feeding, even though adverse reactions in these conditions have not been reported. On the contrary, they have been used successfully in some patients both during pregnancy and lactation without any detrimental effect on mother or baby; as recently reported.

The concentration of bisphosphonates in extraosseous cells is extremely low, which explains the lack of toxicity.

Bisphosphonates Currently Used in Osteoporosis

Only oral bisphosphonates have been approved so far:

▶ Alendronate (Fosamax) 10 mg daily orally or 70 mg once weekly orally (Fosamax once weekly 70 mg)
▶ Risedronate (Actonel) 5 mg daily orally or 35 mg once weekly orally (Actonel once weekly 35 mg)
▶ Etidronate (e.g., Didronel) 400 mg daily orally for 14 days every 3 months

Alendronate

This aminobisphosphonate has been tested in clinical trials involving more than 17,000 patients, and it has been prescribed for about 4 million patients in 80 different countries world-wide. It has been approved for treatment of postmenopausal osteoporosis as well as cortisone-induced and involutional bone loss in both men and women.

Alendronate 10 mg orally for 1–3 years resulted in an increase of bone density of 5%–9% compared to the control group – only calcium and vitamin D. After the first year of alendronate therapy, the vertebral fracture rate was reduced by 59%, and the hip fracture rate by 63% after 18 months. Significant increases in bone density were seen after 3 months of therapy and the success rate was 95% after 1 year. Moreover, as shown by the FIT study ("Fracture Intervention Trial") many patients reported decreases in pain and morbidity. Alendronate achieved significant decreases in fracture rates of vertebrae, hip, and forearm. Similar results were reported in men and in patients with cortisone-induced osteoporosis. The results have been confirmed by several large international trials.

Alendronate 5 mg orally daily has also been approved for prevention of osteoporosis. Because of the low side effects, 5 mg alendronate daily is especially useful in women who do not take HRT for whatever reason.

A recent study has shown that combining HRT and alendronate therapy results in a significantly greater increase in BMD compared to either oestrogen or alendronate alone.

A significant advance in therapy has been the development of the *alendronate once weekly dose of 70 mg*. Numerous animal and clinical studies have shown that alendronate given once weekly as a single tablet produces less irritation of the oesophageal mucosa. Pharmacological studies have also shown that 0.5%–1% is absorbed of which 50% is deposited on the resorptive surfaces of bone, where it inhibits the osteoclasts. The same local concentration of alendronate is achieved by daily as by weekly intake. Similarly, the rate of increase in bone density was also equal after daily or weekly administration. Moreover, bone remodelling – i.e., resorption and formation – were also identical. A most important aspect of the once weekly dosage is that patient acceptance, compliance, and tolerance are greatly increased. In the *first head-to-head trial*, the efficacy of alendronate and risedronate have been compared. In this study, alendronate 70 mg once weekly produced significantly greater BMD increases at the spine and all hip sites over 12 months than did risedronate 5 mg daily. These differences may be due to the antiresorptive efficacy of alendronate 70 mg once weekly as opposed to reduced bioavailability of risedronate resulting from postmeal dosing, or both.

The once weekly dosage of modern bisphosphonates has increased compliance and avoids possible gastrointestinal side effects.

Risedronate

This bisphosphonate has also been tested in large clinical trials involving 15,000 patients. At a daily oral dose of 5 mg, the results were similar to those obtained by alendronate, with the exception of the femoral neck. Significant differences occurred only in one subgroup. Risedronate is well tolerated even by patients with gastrointestinal problems. It is effective in cortisone-induced osteoporosis and has been approved in the USA and in Europe for treatment of postmenopausal osteoporosis. Risedronate 35 mg and 50 mg once a week provide the same efficacy and safety as the daily 5 mg regimen. Therefore, the lower dose, *35 mg risedronate once a week*, is considered to be the optimal dosage for women with postmenopausal osteoporosis. Meanwhile, results of a 5-year, placebo-controlled clinical experience have demonstrated that the long-term efficacy and the beneficial effects of risedronate treatment are sustained over a 3 year period.

Etidronate

This first generation bisphosphonate is the only one which is administered intermittently. It is given daily 400 mg for 2 weeks every 3 months. No food or drink may be taken before or after the ingestion of the tablet. Calcium 500 mg daily is taken after the etidronate and the cycle is repeated after 3 months. However, etidronate is being replaced by the newer aminobisphosphonates as described above.

Etidronate – no longer first choice!

Ibandronate

This bisphosphonate is currently being tested in large-scale placebo-controlled trials. In a previous placebo-controlled trial testing oral ibandronate, the optimal daily dose was shown to be 2.5 mg, which resulted in increases in bone density of up to 10 % after 2 years. This progress has been achieved due to increases in the potency of the drug and improvements in the methods of administration – oral or intravenous. The following *treatment regimens* have significantly reduced vertebral fracture risk by about 50 %–65 % after 3 years:

Ibandronate is currently being tested for intermittent (weeks or months) oral and intravenous administration.

▶ Oral daily 2.5 mg
▶ Oral once weekly 25 mg
▶ Oral intermittent (20 mg every other day for 12 doses every 3 months = ca. 1 month per trimester)
▶ Intravenous every 3 months 2 mg (bolus or infusion).

A reduction in the risk of nonvertebral fractures (69 %) was observed in patients receiving daily ibandronate who had low femoral neck BMD (T-score $<$–3 SD). Ibandronate therapy also produced significant increases in BMD and sustained suppression of biochemical markers of bone turnover. All regimens noted above were well tolerated with an overall safety profile similar to placebo. The results of these randomised studies indicate that the efficacy of ibandronate depends on the total oral or intravenous dose given rather than on the dosing schedule. New, flexible dosing regimens such as once monthly will improve convenience and lead to enhanced patient compliance.

Ibandronate was also effective in secondary osteoporosis (e. g., Klinefelter's syndrome and glucocorticoid-induced osteoporosis) as well as osteoporosis in men. For *prevention* of osteoporosis, longer intervals between infusions – even 1 year instead of 3 months – are also being tested.

The progress of ibandronate has been achieved due to increases in the potency of the drug and improvements in the methods of administration – oral or intravenous.

Clodronate, Pamidronate, Zoledronate, and Neridronate

These bisphosphonates have long been approved for treatment of hypercalcemia and when osteolyses are present, though lower doses are used. Since these bisphosphonates are not yet authorised for use in osteoporosis, they should only be prescribed in collaboration with a responsible medical centre and after the patient's informed consent has been obtained. Clinical studies of zoledronate in osteoporosis are now in progress, including a trial of an annual injection for prevention.

The Intravenous Approach

A possible significant development in bisphosphonate therapy is the current trial of an annual injection for prevention of osteoporosis.

Intravenous therapy has gained a high degree of compliance, especially with patients who are already taking a number of other drugs. Additional advantages are 100 % bioavailability and no gastrointestinal side effects. Moreover, the effects on bone density and fracture rate are comparable to those of oral therapy. The following dosages and time intervals are currently used:

Clodronate (Ostac, Lodronat, Bonefos)   600 mg infusion every 3 months
Pamidronate (Aredia)   30 mg infusion every 3 months
Ibandronate (Bondronat)   2 mg infusion or injection every 3 months
Zoledronate (Zometa)   4 mg infusion every 6–12 months

Administration of bisphosphonates at intervals of 3 months is based on the observation that a single intravenous dose inhibits bone re-

sorption for many weeks. It should be stressed that these bisphosphonates have not yet been officially approved for treatment of osteoporosis and they should be only given in recognised centres and after obtaining the patients' written consent.

The optimal *duration* of bisphosphonate therapy is 1–3 years,
depending on the severity of osteoporosis and the increase in bone
density. Three phases are recognised:

The optimal duration
of bisphosphonate therapy
is 1–3 years.

- ▶ Repair (up to 12 months)
- ▶ Rebuilding (6–36 months)
- ▶ Maintenance (24–60 months)

The highest rate of increase in bone density occurs during the first
12 months when the resorption lacunae are repaired and refilled with
bone. It is thought that this repair of the trabecular bone during the
first year of therapy is responsible for the reduction of the fracture rate
which could not be attributed only to the increased bone density.
Duing the rebuilding and maintenance phases, the increase is less because during these periods the trabecular structure and width are being restored. After 1–3 years of treatment, results of annual measurements of BMD will determine when bisphosphonate therapy should
be resumed. Some studies have already shown that the positive effect
on mineral density of both cortical and trabecular bone is maintained
for one year after cessation of bisphosphonate therapy. While immediate bone loss was seen after withdrawal of oestrogen therapy, this was
not the case after withdrawal of alendronate or combination therapy.
The assumption that an increase in bone density under bisphosphonate therapy requires addition of fluorides is false.

Long-term Follow-up Studies

Previous fears of a "frozen, poor-quality bisphosphonate bone" have
not been confirmed. Clinical studies of alendronate conducted over
more than 7 years have demonstrated the following:

- ▶ Over a period of 3 years, approximately 70 mg of alendronate were
  incorporated into the bones. With such a minute amount of bisphosphonate when the skeleton contains 2,000,000 mg of hydroxyapatite, physicochemical damage is practically excluded. The

same holds true for the other modern bisphosphonates. Moreover, disturbances of mineralisation are no longer seen.

Long-term follow-up studies, now over 10 years, have not revealed any detrimental effects of bisphosphonates on bone: no relevant increase in microcracks, no decrease in mineralisation, no deterioration of cortical or trabecular structure.

▶ Due to reduced turnover, the mean tissue age of bone is increased with bisphosphonate therapy, as is bone mineralisation. Increased mineralisation under bisphosphonate treatment affects a number of biochemical properties of bone: stiffness is increased, while ultimate displacement is decreased. This shift towards higher mineralisation in bone tissue might also decrease fracture risk.

▶ After 7 years of therapy with alendronate and 5 years of therapy with risedronate, the bone mass still increased by about 1% a year, indicating that basic remodelling with a positive bone balance remains unchanged. Meanwhile, the effect of oral alendronate after 10 years of follow up has been published. Alendronate treatment was effective and well tolerated for 10 years. Discontinuation after 5 years of treatment resulted in only gradual, not accelerated bone loss during 5 years of follow up. Continuous treatment with the recommended 10 mg daily dose yielded sustained beneficial effects on bone density and remodelling, with no indication that the efficacy was reduced.

▶ Bone biopsy findings have shown that after 7 years of therapy with alendronate the trabecular architecture and lamellar structure remained unchanged and microfractures were not found. At present, there is no evidence that microdamage accumulation occurs during treatment with clinical doses of bisphosphonates.

▶ The number of normal hydroxyapatite crystals increased, thereby rendering bone more resistant to compression. In contrast, fluoro-apatite crystals, which are incorporated into the mineral phase of bone during fluoride poisoning, though denser than hydroxyapatite, are brittle and shatter easily.

Monitoring the Effects of Bisphosphonates

The following parameters can be used to estimate *success of therapy*:

▶ Decrease in collagen breakdown products and tartrate resistant acid phosphatase (TRAP) in urine and/or serum
▶ Increase in biochemical markers of bone formation
▶ Increase in BMD (DEXA of lumbar spine and hip)
▶ Decrease in fracture rate (vertebral and extravertebral)

▶ Decrease in osteoporotic bone pain
▶ Increase in quality of life and mobility
▶ Decrease in duration of hospitalisation

After approximately 3–6 weeks of therapy there should be a decrease in the biochemical markers of bone resorption. If, after 2–3 months of therapy markers of resorption have not decreased by about 30 %–40 % and markers of bone formation increased by 20 %–30 %, then the patient should be interviewed and the method of taking the bisphosphonate investigated. Subjective parameters such as pain, mobility, and quality of life are only considered as secondary criteria. Bone mineral density should be measured annually during therapy with bisphosphonate. A recent review of drug treatments for postmenopausal osteoporosis has confirmed the positive effects of bisphosphonates as demonstrated in bone biopsies.

It should be remembered that different therapies effect bone remodelling and bone quality/strength in different ways, so that, for example, bone structure may be changed and bone fragility decreased without necessarily a significant increase in BMD.

Another important aspect of osteoporosis therapy is: what happens when therapy is discontinued? Results of a randomised, double blind, placebo-controlled trial which addressed this question have recently been published: accelerated bone loss was seen after withdrawal of oestrogen therapy (2 years) but not after combination therapy (oestrogen and alendronate) for 2 years, or alendronate alone for 2 years. These data should obviously be considered when therapy in postmenopausal women is planned. These results also provide evidence in support of the probable efficacy of a single annual injection of potent bisphosphonates (for example zoledronate or ibandronate) for prevention and therapy of postmenopausal and involutional osteoporosis.

Various parameters are in use to monitor short- and long-term effects of therapy. The most important endpoint is, of course, decrease in risk and rate of fracture.

BMD should be measured annually during therapy with bisphosphonate.

Nonresponders to Bisphosphonates: Do They Exist?

Should there be no increase in BMD after 1 year as indicated by DXA measurement, five possibilities should be considered:

▶ Medication was not taken: telopeptides (markers of bone resorption) should be checked.

If there is no response to oral and intravenous administration, a primary disorder may be the cause of the osteoporosis.

▶ Medication was not taken according to instructions: discussion with patient for information and clarification.

▶ Possible "nonabsorber" and therefore "nonresponder": change to intravenous administration of nitrogen-containing bisphosphonates.

▶ An undiagnosed primary malignant disorder may be present: Investigation including MRI and bone biopsy must be carried out.

CHAPTER 15 Raloxifene: A Potent Selective Oestrogen Receptor Modulator (SERM)

A Brief Survey of SERMs: New Selective Antiresorptive Agents

In the last decade, more and more oestrogen-like substances have been developed and introduced. These drugs bind to the oestrogen receptors (ERs α and β) throughout the body. For example, *tamoxifen* has long been given to women with a history of breast cancer. It acts as an oestrogen antagonist on breast tissue but as an oestrogen on other organs and tissues in the body namely bone, liver, and fat. Tamoxifen inhibits growth of any residual breast cancer cells remaining in the body if they still have oestrogen receptors.

Raloxifene: Utilisation of Physiological Effects on Bone

The positive effect on bone has been further developed in the SERM of the second generation called *raloxifene*, which has no effect on breast or uterus. Raloxifene was originally investigated as a treatment for breast cancer. Uterine bleeding, breast tenderness, and water retention are not observed with raloxifene. However, "hot flashes" and leg cramps occurred in about 30 % of previously asymptomatic patients, as raloxifene blocks all oestrogen receptors remaining in the body and thereby also the effects of the small amount of oestrogen that might still be produced. Leg cramps, especially nocturnal, can be treated by supplements of magnesium, which is freely available. An international clinical trial, the *Multiple Outcomes of Raloxifene Evaluation* (MORE) study, has shown that the risk of a vertebral body fracture in patients taking raloxifene is half that of a control group. After 3 years, raloxifene 60 mg daily increased BMD by 2 %–3 % at the hips and spine and reduced the risk of new fractures by 30 %–50 %. New clinical ver-

A woman may take oestrogen for the first few years of menopause until the flashes are controlled and then switch to raloxifene.

Fig. 15.1. Mechanisms of action of raloxifene on osteoblast, osteoclast, and osteocyte

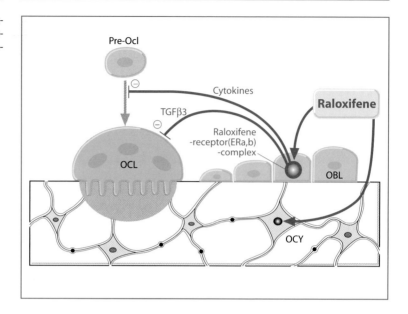

tebral fractures were reduced by 68% after 1 year treatment with raloxifene. The risk of breast cancer is significantly reduced (60%–70%) in women taking raloxifene. This effect was mainly due to a 90% reduction of oestrogen-receptor-positive breast cancer. The Raloxifene Use for The Heart (RUTH) trial is further evaluating this positive effect.

The SERMs have tremendous potential for reducing a variety of chronic diseases in women associated with ageing.

The SERMs action exert their effects by binding with high affinity to the oestrogen receptors (ERs) of which two different subtypes have so far been identified (ER-α and ER-β). These receptor subtypes appear throughout the body with a predominance of ER-α expression in the reproductive tissues and a predominance of ER-β expression in nonreproductive tissues. The structural features of each SERM differ, so that unique ligand-induced changes take place in the ERs which are thought to be the likely basis for tissue-selective pharmacology. For example, raloxifene operates as an oestrogen agonist in bone but as an antagonist in the breast and uterus. The mechanism by which SERMs inhibit bone resorption is likely to be the same as the oestrogen mechanism, that is, by blocking production of cytokines that promote osteoclast differentiation and by stimulating TGF-β3, which suppresses osteoclast activation. TGF β3 also decreases expression of IL-6, which stimulates bone resorption. Raloxifene probably also acts on osteocytes, which participate in control of bone remodelling. This physiological mode of action leads to a completely normal bone structure without mineralisation defects or increased numbers of microcracks. Studies of the pharmacokinetics of SERMs have shown considerable differences in their bioavailability. Hepatic, but not renal impairment affects their metabolism and there is a possibility of interaction with other agents such as warfarin and aromatase inhibitors.

In summary, SERMs now constitute a new approach to therapy and have been approved for prevention and treatment of postmenopausal osteoporosis while decreasing the risks of cardiac and circulatory disorders without the unwanted side-effects and risks associated with hormone replacement therapy. In a recent study, SERMs have also been tried in men and the results are expected soon. Recommended dosage: 60 mg raloxifene (Evista, Optruma) orally daily, without restrictions as to when, and preferably with supplements of vitamin D and calcium. Raloxifene is the treatment of choice for postmenopausal women, especially those

Raloxifene is most useful in women of middle menopausal age (55–65 years).

▶ With high risk for breast cancer or cardiovascular diseases
▶ With high risk of vertebral fracture
▶ With modest degrees of osteopenia in the middle menopausal period (age 55–65)
▶ With osteoporosis diagnosed by DXA in the middle menopausal period (age 55–65)

Raloxifene substantially reduce the risk of breast cancer.

Present osteoporotic therapy inhibits bone resorption. The search is on for effective stimulants of bone formation. There are many possible candidates, some already tested, other in process.

All currently available and approved drugs for therapy of osteoporosis inhibit bone resorption. By reducing the activity of the osteoclast, they all have the capacity to increase BMD and to reduce fracture risk. Despite their great value, the antiresorptives are generally not associated with dramatic increases in bone density or with production of new bone. Reduction of fracture risk, although highly significant, is rarely more than 50 % of the baseline risk. Another approach is osteoanabolic therapy, with stimulation of new bone formation. Fluoride, strontium, GH, insulin-like growth factor, the statins, and PTH are the main candidates.

Osteoanabolic Action:
Paradoxical Effects Depend on Type of Administration

One advantage is that parathyroid hormone fragments are quickly cleared by the body and are not incorporated into the bone. Their action is very short-lived.

Parathormone (PTH). This hormone is a principal regulator of calcium homeostasis and was developed millions of years ago when mammals moved from the calcium-rich ocean to a calcium-poor, land-based diet. It is a polypeptide with 84 amino acids. PTH stimulates release of calcium and phosphate from bone and synthesis of active vitamin D in the kidney. This in turn promotes calcium transport in the gastrointestinal tract. But when given intermittently by injection, PTH stimulates osteoblasts and new bone formation on all available osseous surfaces, while the number of osteoclasts and bone resorption remain unchanged. PTH has been shown to increase bone density, strength, and connectivity. However, the underlying molecular physiology accounting for the true anabolic effect of PTH remains unknown. It is also unknown why intermittent low dose PTH administration differs so dramatically from continuous administration in its effect on bone cells. Recently, evidence has emerged that PTH reduces osteoblast apoptosis, prolonging osteoblast survival and potentiating its function of collagen synthesis. Studies on bone biopsies have confirmed these findings. Biopsies were taken before and after 18–36 months of therapy with PTH in both men and women. Results showed that PTH stimulates remodelling, resulting in an increased percentage of newly formed matrix but of lower mineral density . This would indicate that calcium and vitamin D supplements are required together with PTH.

The combination of PTH with calcitriol strengthens its anabolic effect and induces an increase of 10%–30% in bone density after 1–2 years of treatment. The fracture rate is also significantly decreased. In one study PTH (1–34-hPTH) was given subcutaneously as a daily injection of 500 IU for 1 year. In another trial hPTH(1–34) was given i.m. once a week with similar results. Back pain, nausea, and headache were the most common side-effects, but these occurred infrequently and in a dose-dependent manner. Less than 5% of the patients showed increased serum calcium levels, but they were asymptomatic. Moreover, there have been no cases of osteogenic sarcomas, and it is reasonable to assume that PTH is safe in humans for short-term administration.

Combinations with oestrogens also appear promising and are currently under investigation in clinical trials. The data obtained so far make two important points:

▶ PTH plus oestrogen has a greater effect on bone mass than either alone.
▶ Combination therapy has beneficial effects in both the spine and the femur, the two most vulnerable areas for subsequent fractures.

It has already been shown that the combination of the anabolic PTH with raloxifene is promising. Patients treated with raloxifene showed a rapid response to PTH. However, results of recent trials with the combination of PTH and alendronate in postmenopausal women showed no evidence of synergy between PTH and the bisphosphonate. There was even an indication that the simultaneous administration of these two drugs reduced the stimulatory effects of PTH on bone formation. Nevertheless, other preliminary studies have demonstrated that timing is crucial and that sequential administration, i.e., PTH followed by a bisphosphonate or by raloxifene, might be effective and beneficial. New analogues of PTH and of "PTH related peptide" are also being tested. A new PTH receptor ("PTH2 receptor") has recently

Simultaneous administration of PTH with a bisphosphonate inhibits the stimulation of bone formation by PTH.

been described. Results of more studies now underway are awaited with interest.

PTH as an anabolic therapy for osteoporosis will soon play a major role, but some questions remain to be answered:

PTH as an osteoanabolic agent is especially valuable for patients with severe osteoporosis.

▶ Which patients are most likely to benefit from PTH?
▶ Is PTH only indicated in severe osteoporosis, with presence of fractures?
▶ How long should patients receive PTH?
▶ Is it better to treat with a combination of PTH plus an antiresorptive agent or PTH alone?
▶ What is the best sequence for combination therapy?
▶ Is there a more rapid response to PTH when pretreated with raloxifene?
▶ What is the mechanism of PTH's anabolic action on bone?

Calcitonin and Fluoride: No Longer First Line Therapy

Calcitonin is a polypeptide hormone produced by the parafollicular C cells of the thyroid. It inhibits the osteoclasts by binding to specific receptors on the cell surface. Calcitonin can be given as a subcutaneous injection or in a nasal spray. However use of calcitonin is limited because of its side effects such as feelings of heat as well as nausea, and mucosal irritation with use of the nasal spray. The most valid indication for calcitonin today is the intractable pain caused by a vertebral fracture, although even here its use is limited because of the superior results of intravenous bisphosphonates. On the other hand, the calcitonins are physiological peptides which can be metabolised and therefore are not retained in the body. Toxic effects have not been reported. Calcitonins are therefore suitable for children and in pregnancy and during breast feeding.

Calcitonin is a potent pain reliever, it works without causing constipation and is very helpful in patients with an acute vertebral fracture. It is also suitable for children and women during pregnancy and breast feeding.

For economic reasons, *fluoride* is still used in some countries for treatment of osteoporosis, but its role in prevention of fractures has not been confirmed in clinical trials. The recommended dose ranges from 20–200 mg sodium fluoride daily (elementary fluoride constitutes half of this amount): There is general agreement that fluoride stimulates osteoblastic bone formation and thereby increases bone mass; however, mechanical resistance of the newly formed bone is poor and it is even liable to fracture easily. Fluoride is incorporated into the crystal in place of the hydroxyl group in hydroxyapatite, thereby changing crystal size and conformation and producing poor quality woven bone. A high dosage of fluoride results in increases in bone density but vertebral fractures are not significantly reduced. Moreover, especially with high doses there are serious adverse reactions:

The use of fluoride to treat osteoporosis has waxed and waned in recent years. Results from clinical trials have not shown a beneficial effect of fluoride in prevention of fractures, though bone mass is increased.

▶ Gastrointestinal side effects: epigastric complaints, vomiting and diarrhoea.

▶ Lower extremity pain syndrome (LEPS): pains in the hips, knees, and ankles. The cause may be delayed microcallus formation in the affected areas of these bones.

▶ Iatrogenic fluorosis: severe cases can be identified on X-rays as overgrowth and thickening of the bone. This may be due to incorrect treatment. The patient sometimes increases the dose without medical advice because of continuing complaints and pain. However, it is not known whether there is an individual tendency to develop fluorosis.

▶ Exostoses and calcium deposits in the ligaments.

Many problems encountered when using fluoride in the treatment of osteoporosis result from its narrow therapeutic window. The toxic threshold for skeletal fluoride is between 0.6% and 0.8% of bone mineral.

The latest clinical trials indicate that much lower doses (e.g., 15 mg daily) should be given over 3–4 years and always together with vitamin D and calcium. It is not known whether intermittent fluoride has any advantages over continuous, and the long-term effects have also not yet been clarified. Slow-release sodium fluoride at a lower dose (50 mg/d) appears to be associated with reduction of fracture risk in one study, but confirmation of these results is not yet available. These and other question will probably be answered when results of the present ongoing studies become available. Because of the various side effects and the availability of other efficacious agents, fluoride treatment is presently not recommended and not approved by the FDA for treatment of osteoporosis.

Other Medications in Use or Under Investigation

Leptin – a central hormone with many functions – is now under intense investigation in osteoporosis.

Leptin. This is a hormone with many diverse functions. It is produced by fat cells, acts as a "saturation hormone," and influences glucose metabolism and the production of sex hormones. It has long been known that sex hormone deficiency stimulates bone resorption while overweight inhibits it. This underlies the speculation that bone mass, body weight, and sexual glands are regulated by a common mechanism in the brain. Attempts are currently under way to influence the level of leptin or its receptors and thereby develop a novel way to treat osteoporosis (see also Chapter 2, pages 20–22).

Growth factors. These are produced primarily by cells in the bone marrow and they regulate the proliferation, function, and interactions of bone cells. There are various regulators of bone formation – such as parathormone, insulin, growth hormone, and cortisone, which all function by stimulation of growth factors in particular bone cells. In one clinical trial, bone formation was increased simply by the administration of one of these factors. It is anticipated that in the not-too distant future individually "tailored" growth hormones will be administered for the different types of osteoporosis. Prostaglandins also modulate metabolism of bone. PGE2 has a distinctly anabolic effect on trabecular bone – presumably by stimulation of proliferation and differentiation of the precursors of osteoblasts.

Most of the systemic hormones probably work by stimulating the production of growth factors, such as insulin-like growth factor (IGF-1) produced by osteoblasts.

Statins. These are given for lowering concentrations of fat and cholesterol in the blood. Women who were treated with statins showed a higher bone density and a lower fracture risk than comparable women who had not been treated with statins. Animal studies have shown that statins shorten the life-span of osteoclasts and thereby inhibit resorption of bone. Should this positive action of statins on bone be confirmed, then statins could become an effective drug for prevention of arteriosclerosis and of osteoporosis. But statins have one disadvantage: they act on the liver and therefore will never replace the bone-specific bisphosphonates in the treatment of osteoporosis, though the mechanism of action of the two drugs is similar. The statins, when administered orally, are almost totally cleared by first pass through the liver. It is also unclear how these agents reach the bone and how they affect bone turnover. It is still unclear how the statins can stimulate bone formation while the bisphophonates, working in the same pathway, inhibit bone resorption. Nevertheless, in the future specific statins selected for their high affinity to bone, may be useful agents for prevention or treatment of osteoporosis. The indications for such agents will be broad if they benefit both the skeleton and the cardiovascular system.

In spite of much speculation, anticipation and investigation, the ability of statins to reduce risk and prevent fractures has not been conclusively demonstrated.

Strontium. In low doses, strontium increases the density of the spongy bone. It reduces resorption and stimulates formation of bone, leading to a gain in bone mass and improved bone mechanical properties. The increment in bone density is comparable to that achieved by fluoride: up to 20%. The decrease in fracture risk will depend on whether the quality of bone is maintained. It is expected that strontium ranelate

Results from early clinical trials with strontium for prevention and treatment of osteoporosis have been very encouraging, but more work is needed on the "quality" of the bone produced.

may have potential value in the prevention and treatment of bone loss. The results of the prevention PREVention Of early postmenopausal loss by Strontiumm ranelate (PREVOS) and the treatment STRontium Administration for Treatment of Osteoporosis (STRATOS) investigations of strontium for the prevention of bone loss and the therapy of osteoporosis have now been published. Strontium was well tolerated; effective doses were 1 g daily for prevention and 2 g daily for therapy. However, in vitro studies have revealed a complicated dose-dependent action of strontium on bone cells and further studies are needed for clarification.

The tetracyclines inhibit bone resorption by inhibition of enzymes and by inducing osteoclast apoptosis.

Tetracyclins (chemically modified tetracyclins, CMTs). These prevent bone resorption by inhibition of matrix metalloproteinases, as well as induction of apoptosis in osteoclasts. The possible applications and the risks of these agents are being tested in clinical trials.

Fractures: No Reason to Despair

Many, if not the majority of fractures occur as a result of falling, and approximately 5% of older people require hospitalisation.

The *most common risk factors for falls* identified in 16 large studies are:

▶ Muscle weakness
▶ History of falls
▶ Impairment of balance and motion
▶ Lack of devices for protection and assistance in walking
▶ Visual impairment or defective eyesight, not well compensated
▶ Arthritis
▶ Psychological factors such as depression
▶ Cognitive impairment
▶ Age >80 years

In the *OFELY-study*, seven independent predictors of fragility fractures in postmenopausal women were identified reflecting different potential mechanisms. In order of decreasing importance, they were:

▶ Previous fragility fractures
▶ Low BMD
▶ Insufficient physical activity
▶ Decreased grip strength
▶ Older age groups
▶ Maternal history of fractures
▶ Patient history of falls

If a patient has had any fracture after age 40 and has a low bone density, his risk of hip fracture may increase fivefold.

---

* In collaboration with Dr. C. Bartl

Note main reasons for falling and try to avoid them wherever and whenever possible.

Table 18.1. Main causes of falls in the elderly

General deterioration
• Poor postural control • Weakness • Abnormal gait • Poor vision • Slow reaction time • Anxiety and agitation • Fear of falling
Specific diseases and drugs
• Cerebrovascular disease • Parkinson's disease • Arthritis • Cataracts and retinal degeneration • Blackouts • Urinary incontinence • Sedatives • Hypotensive drugs • Alcohol
Environmental causes
• Low-level lighting • Slippery surfaces • Uneven pavements • Lack of assist devices in bathrooms • Loose rugs • Bad weather, wind, and rain • Tripping over mats or grandchildren's toys

Your bones are like a bank savings account for calcium. If you have insufficient calcium funds, you may have to pay up with a fracture.

These items should be included in the clinical assessment of risks for osteoporotic fractures in postmenopausal women.

Five main *factors lead to weakening of bone and pathologic fractures*:

▶ Reduced bone mass (density)
▶ Discontinuities in microarchitecture of bone
▶ Disturbance of mineralisation ("osteoporomalacia")
▶ Increased, unregulated bone turnover ("secondary hyperparathyroidism")
▶ Increased tendency to fall

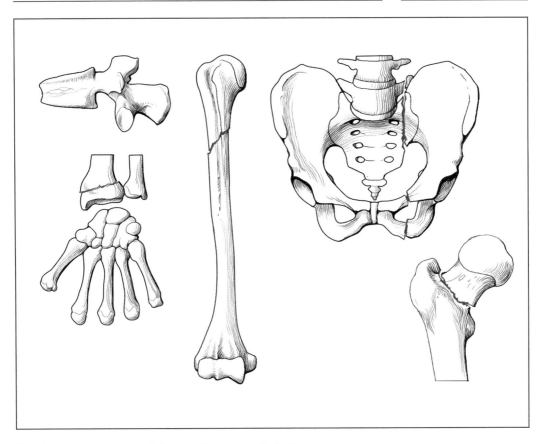

Fig. 18.1. Bone sites commonly involved in osteoporotic fractures

About a third of older persons fall at least once a year, but only about 5% of these falls result in a fracture. Taller and thinner patients are more likely to sustain a fracture on falling than shorter, plumper ones. Wrist fractures usually involve a fall onto an outstretched hand. Therefore, it appears that the orientation of the fall is an important factor in determining the kind of fracture. Forces in the spine or ribs generated by activities such as lifting, stepping down, or coughing may also be sufficient to cause a vertebral or rib fracture. Other factors such as degenerative disc alterations and the distribution of body weight influence biomechanical forces in the spine and thereby the risk of vertebral fractures. The elderly are more liable to fall because of:

Table 18.2. Risk factors for osteoporotic fracture

Nonmodifiable
• Personal history of fracture as an adult • Maternal history of fracture • Caucasian race • Advanced age • Female sex • Late menarche • Dementia • Poor health/frailty
Potentially modifiable
• Current cigarette smoking • Low body weight • Oestrogen deficiency • Testosterone deficiency • Vitamin D deficiency • Low dietary calcium intake • Excess alcohol consumption • Impaired eyesight despite adequate correction • Recurrent falls • Inadequate physical activity • Glucocorticoid therapy • Various medications

Table 18.3. Osseous and extraosseous factors that may affect fracture risk

Skeletal factors: increased bone fragility
• Bone configuration • Bone microarchitecture • Bone density • Bone quality
Extraskeletal factors: increased risk of trauma
• Increased propensity to fall • Environmental hazard • Loss of protective responses

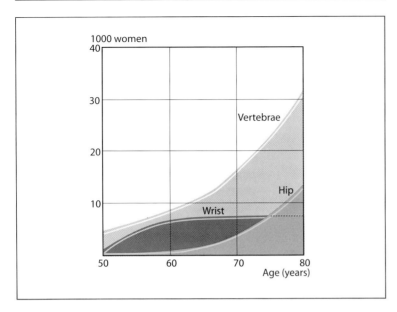

Fig. 18.2. Age-related incidence of osteoporotic fractures

► Reduced muscle mass and strength
► Slowing of reflexes
► Loss of equilibrium
► Impaired vision
► Impaired coordination
► Hypnotics, sedatives, and psychotropics
► Alcohol
► Obstacles such as loose mats, cables, wires, and small pieces of furniture, etc.

Check the workplace and especially the home for possible obstacles and remove or neutralise them.

Fractures of the wrist or vertebrae are early manifestations of postmenopausal osteoporosis, while hip fractures are more common in the late stage of age-related osteoporosis. Generally, the lower the bone mass, the less trauma is necessary to cause a fracture, which is why a fracture of a rib or vertebra can be sustained after coughing or rolling over in bed. The risk of fractures for the rest of their lives in 50-year-old women and men (in brackets) are:

Proximal femur	18%	(6%)
Vertebral column	16%	(5%)
Distal radius	15%	(3%)
Any location	40%	(13%)

One year after a hip fracture, patients were found to have a 5–9% loss of bone and muscle mass, even in the face of adequate calcium intake. Consequently, many never become independent or walk as well again.

In the course of a life-time women lose 35%–50% of the trabecular bone and 25%–30% of the compact bone. If an osteoporosis-associated fracture has occurred, the following steps should be taken:

▶ Alleviate the pain
▶ Accelerate fracture healing by appropriate surgical, nonoperative, and other supportive measures
▶ Restore mobility as quickly as possible
▶ Exercise the muscles
▶ Prevent future fractures
▶ Improve bone mass and skeletal stability
▶ Nerve root injections given patients locally before operative or other therapy are effective in reducing pain

Rehabilitation. This is indicated in patients with manifest osteoporosis and it may last for months, but usually no longer than a year. Each patient should receive guidance as outlined previously.

Management of Osteoporotic Fractures

Physical therapeutic programmes should consist of:
• Measures to prevent falls
• Management of complications secondary to falls
• Management of chronic pain to decrease immobility and risk of fall

The goals of orthopaedic treatment of osteoporosis are rapid mobilisation and a return to normal activities – in other words rapid and aggressive management to avoid undesirable consequences.

General guidelines for the management of osteoporotic fractures are:

▶ Elderly patients are best treated by rapid fracture management aimed at early restoration of mobility. In addition, the extent of the operative intervention should be minimised in order to reduce operative time, blood loss, and stress to the patient. Indeed, a delay of more than two days before operative intervention proved to be an important predictor of mortality within one year of the time of the fracture.
▶ The goal of operative intervention is to achieve stable fracture fixation and to return to a full weight-bearing status.

▶ The primary cause of failure of internal fixation is the inability of the osteoporotic bone to support fixation devices.

▶ Although fracture healing proceeds normally in almost all osteoporotic patients, an inadequate calcium and vitamin D intake can result in deficits in remodelling or in callus mineralisation. Therefore, for optimal results calcium, vitamin D, and protein supplementation should be administered in the peri- and postoperative periods. The bisphosphonates currently in use and raloxifene have not shown any negative effect on fracture healing.

Fracture Sites and Their Clinical Significance

Osteoporosis only causes symptoms when there is a fracture. It is important to realise that bone loss itself does not cause pain or disability. Hip, spine, and wrist fractures are the most common, although fractures in other parts of the skeleton also occur, particularly in the pelvis, ribs, and humerus. Although any fracture can have a devastating impact on the affected individual, hip fractures are by far the most important from the public health perspective.

Fifty percent of women who are 50 are expected to have some type of fracture due to osteoporosis during their lifetime. Most could be prevented!

Hip Fractures

Hip fractures account for most of the medical costs, being responsible for about 65% of the total costs for osteoporotic fracture. More than 300,000 patients annually in the USA alone sustain a *fracture of the proximal femur*; 25% are men, the average age is around 80 years. One out of every six Caucasian women (15%) will suffer a hip fracture in her lifetime. There are three types of hip fractures: *intertrochanteric*, *femoral neck* and *subcapital*. Fractures of the femoral neck, also called "cervical hip fractures," constitute about a half of all fractures of the proximal femur, and two third of them are displaced. The mean age is now 81 years and half of the patients live alone. Hip fractures are rare below 50 years of age. In more than 90% of patients, hip fractures are caused by fall, and the type of fracture depends on several factors, including the angle and type of fall as well as the patient's neuromuscular and protective responses to the impact. Hip fractures have very serious consequences, most require operative intervention and the patients are frequently left with a disability:

Fig. 18.3. Types of femoral fractures

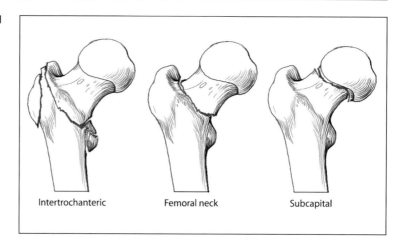

Intertrochanteric   Femoral neck   Subcapital

Fig. 18.4. Surgical repair of hip fractures

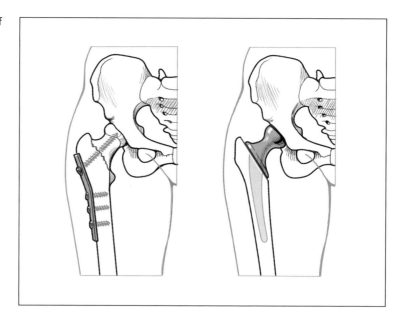

▶ Nearly 20 % of individuals experiencing a hip fracture will die within the first year.
▶ Nearly 25 % require a long-term nursing facility or in-home care.
▶ Nearly 50 % of patients with hip fractures never fully recover their mobility.

Risk factors for the first hip fracture have been well characterised, and include:

▶ Previous fracture at any site
▶ Advanced age
▶ Low body weight
▶ Low bone mineral density

Various treatments are available to reduce fracture risk, but only about 5 % of women are treated properly after the occurrence of the first hip fracture with the intention of avoiding another one.

About 20 % of beds in the orthopaedic wards are still occupied by patients with femoral neck fractures. The surgery depends on the type of fracture. 20 % of patients with type II osteoporosis will suffer from avascular necrosis of the proximal femur. Therefore, implantation of a total endoprosthesis is preferred; it also enables early mobilisation. During rehabilitation special attention must be paid to:

▶ Coordination of movement
▶ Muscle training
▶ Avoidance of risks of tripping and falling

Hip fractures are nearly always painful and require hospitalisation and *surgery*. If the ends of fractures bone are not displaced, the usual treatment is stabilisation of the fracture with a metal plate and pins; however, if the fracture is displaced hip replacement with a prosthesis is often performed. Repair of a femoral neck fracture may take 4–8 months. While healing from a bone fracture it is particularly important to ensure adequate calcium and vitamin D. Studies have shown a 10 % skeletal-wide bone loss following fractures of the long bones, especially of the lower extremities.

From the viewpoint of medical cost and public health, hip fractures are the most important type of fractures.

50 % of hip fracture victims will be incapacitated, 25 % will require long-term nursing home care and about 20 % die within one year from complications. Only one in three will fully recover.

Spinal Fractures

Spinal fractures are more insidious, may even be unrecognised and vary greatly in their manifestations. They may be caused by common activities of everyday living such as bending, lifting, turning, stretching and coughing.

Vertebral fractures are often asymptomatic and not diagnosed. Indeed, only about one third of the vertebral fractures seen on spine radiographs come to clinical attention. Their diagnosis requires lateral radiographs of both the thoracic and the lumbar spine. Vertebral fractures are very common in older women. They are found on radiographs in 5%–10% of women at 55 years, rising to 30%–40% by 80 years. The cortical shell of a vertebral body contributes only about 10% of the resistance to compressive load. Thinning and microcracks in trabecular bone, however. occur with age. Although these heal with callus, excess accumulation of microcracks results in critical weakening, which then leads to vertebral compression fractures. Spine fractures may result from falling, but more commonly they occur spontaneously as a result of coughing, lifting, bending, or turning. Vertebral fractures occur in a heterogeneous set of circumstances, but approximately 50% of vertebral fractures can not be attributed to a known loading activity. Vertebral fractures most commonly involve the mid-thoracic area (T7–T8) and the thoracolumbar junction (T12–L1). In contrast, fractures of the upper thoracic spine (T2–T6) are more likely to be caused by metastatic disease or by multiple myeloma. MRI may help to distinguish malignant from nonmalignant diseases; however, it cannot distinguish between traumatic and osteoporotic fractures.

Spinal fractures typically cause changes in height and shape of the body.

The *symptoms* that are caused by fractures of the spine vary greatly. Some patients experience very little or no pain when the fracture occurs, whereas others feel severe pain. The reason for this difference is not known. Although some affected individuals become pain-free after a few months, others may be left with lasting pain or discomfort. Patients with vertebral fractures experience reinforcement of pain during physical activity such as bending, standing, and rising from bed. Spinal fractures do not usually cause back pain radiating down the legs, which is more typical of radiculopathy caused by disk problems. As a result of changes in body shape (expansion of the waistline and prominence of the abdomen), many patients have trouble finding clothes that fit. Garments fitted at the waist can no longer be worn. The long-term effects of vertebral fractures are still underestimated: many result in chronic back pain and limitation of activities. Multiple vertebral fractures can deform the thorax and seriously restrict pulmonary function.

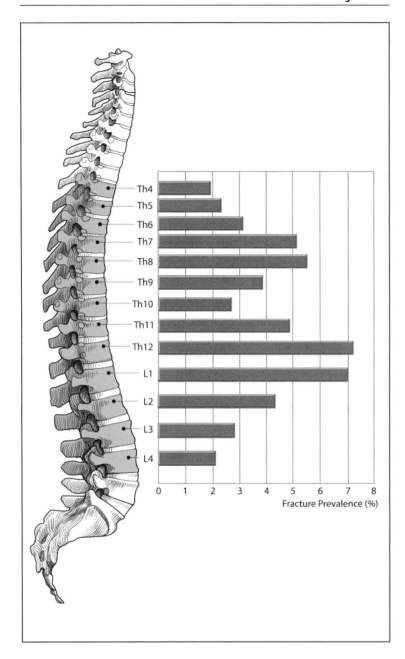

Fig. 18.6. Restoration of vertebral shape by injection of bone cement (vertebro- or kyphoplasty)

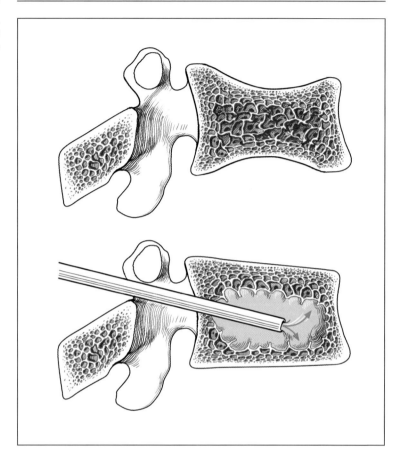

During the phase of repair, attention must be given to restoration of muscle strength and mobility and prevention of progression of osteoporosis by antiresorptive therapy and supplements.

The *repair phase* lasts 2–4 months, during which the use of orthopaedic appliances and corsets should be kept to as short a time as possible. Their purpose is alleviation of pain and avoidance of kyphosis and of reduced lung function. Specialised bandages and supports may be utilised according to the instructions of the orthopaedic specialist. Rehabilitative strategies which increase the strength of spinal muscles in bearing loads across the spine will reduce the load on vertebral bodies and thereby decrease the risk of fracture in mechanically incompetent bone. Research into the risk of vertebral fractures found that a 2 SD decrease in lumbar spine BMD gives a four- to sixfold increase in the risk of a new vertebral fracture. One symptomatic vertebral fracture gives a twofold increase in hip fracture, and 2 or more vertebral fractures results in a 12-fold increase in new vertebral fractures.

New technologies in spine surgery are *kyphoplasty* and *vertebroplasty* for the treatment of painful osteoporotic compression fractures that do not respond to conventional treatment. Vertebroplasty is the percutaneous injection of polymethylmethacrylate (PMMA) through one or two bone biopsy needles into the fractured vertebra. After hardening, the PMMA then stabilises the restructured vertebral body. Kyphoplasty involves inserting a bone tamp/balloon into the vertebral body under image guidance. When inflated with PMMA and radiocontrast medium (for visualisation), the bone tamp compacts the cancellous bone, re-expands the vertebral body and elevates the endplates. Both techniques have a high acceptance and use rate. Unilateral transpendicular augmentation is less time consuming than the bilateral procedure and would be preferable if it provided the same mechanical support as the bilateral procedure.

There is 95 % improvement in pain and significant improvement in function following treatment by either of these percutaneous techniques. Kyphoplasty improves height of the fractured vertebra, and improves kyphosis by over 50 %, if performed 3 months from the onset of the fracture. If the procedure is performed after 3 months, height improvement is not as marked. Complications occur with both and relate to cement leakage in both, though less in kyphoplasty in which the cement is confined within the balloon. Cement emboli may occur in vertebroplasty. There is also a potential for significant complications from both procedures: pulmonary, gastrointestinal, vascular, and spinal cord and cauda equina injuries.

Modern therapy of compression fractures aims at restoration of vertebral shape and height by PMMA (a cement-like substance), which is injected into the vertebral bodies (vertebro- and kyphoplasty).

These procedures are effective when performed early, but significant complications can occur.

Wrist Fractures

Colles' fracture (after the Irish surgeon who first described them) is the most frequent fracture before the age of 75 years, occurring mainly in women around menopause. Wrist fractures are painful and require outpatient treatment at the hospital, though more elderly patients may need to be hospitalised. The fractured ends of the bone(s) are sometimes displaced and must be manipulated into place before a cast or splint is put on to stabilise the fracture ends. A fracture of the radius in patients between 40–60 years of age is always a sign of osteoporosis, and calls for immediate measurement of bone density. A

Wrist fractures, though mainly caused by accidental falls, indicate urgent need for BMD measurement especially in women 40-60 years of age.

cast is required for 6–8 weeks, during which time active and passive exercises of the fingers, the hand, the upper arm, and the shoulder should be carried out regularly to preserve their motility and function. A significant complication may arise in the form of algodystrophy. In these patients, there is often persistent pain, tenderness, swelling, and stiffness of the hand that may last many years after the injury.

Humerus Fractures

Three types of humeral fractures occur in osteoporotic patients: fractures of the proximal humerus, the humeral diaphysis, and the supracondylar region of the elbow. These fractures usually result from minor falls and mostly occur with minimal displacement. Fractures of the proximal humerus are common and account for approximately 5 % of fractures of this patient population. Eighty percent of these fractures occur through the cancellous bone of the humeral neck, without significant displacement. These fractures are considered stable and can be treated with immobilisation in a sling. In most cases humeral shaft fractures are also treated by nonoperative methods. Occasionally intramedullary nailing is needed to control angulation. Fractures of the distal humerus with an intra-articular component, however, present a particular challenge to orthopaedic treatment. These fractures are associated with a high degree of morbidity, and elbow stiffness is not uncommon.

Other Fractures

Other fractures occur especially in parts of bones with a large component of trabecular bone.

They include pelvic, distal tibia, or fibula, and rib fractures. At each of these bone sites, there is predominance of trabecular bone. Fractures about the knee (supracondylar fractures of the distal femur or fractures of the tibial plateau) carry a high risk for postoperative degenerative joint disease and arthrofibrosis.

The National Osteoporosis Foundation has established *guiding principles for the treatment of patients with osteoporotic fractures:*

▶ All patients presenting a low-energy hip fracture should be considered as having primary or secondary osteoporosis.

▶ All patients should be placed on 800 IU of vitamin D and 1,200 to 1,500 mg of elemental calcium (preferably calcium citrate) daily.

▶ Before discharge, all patients should be started on alendronate (70 mg per week), risedronate (35 mg per week), or a modern intravenous bisphosphonate (every 3 months). Intravenous administration is the route of choice if the patient has a history of gastrointestinal dysfunction.

▶ Within 6 weeks after discharge, all patients should undergo a DXA scan and a metabolic workup to rule out secondary causes of osteoporosis. For monitoring, a DXA scan should be performed every year.

Improving Quality of Life After Osteoporotic Fractures

Because osteoporosis is a serious and a world-wide problem, we must focus not only on prevention and treatment but also on ways to deal with the results and social consequences of the disease, like pain, depression, loss of self-esteem, and social isolation:

▶ Acute pain can be treated with bed rest for 2–3 days, analgesics, heating pads, massage, and back support.

▶ Chronic pain treatment includes strengthening back extensor muscles with an exercise program and/or weight-bearing activities including walking that improve balance and strengthen back support.

▶ Gait-assisting devices, including canes and walkers, can prevent the osteoporotic patient from falling.

▶ Patients with osteoporotic fractures may often feel anxious, helpless, and depressed due to lifestyle limitations and changes in appearance. Physical advice may help them function independently at home, and support groups bring patients together and provide useful information.

As in all chronic disorders, early diagnosis and treatment are important in osteoporosis. It is much easier and cheaper to prevent fractures than to try to regain use after a bone has broken.

The foundations for improvement of the quality of life in patients after osteoporotic fracture are threefold:
- Fast, efficient and successful treatment of the fractures
- Restoration and maintenance of mobility
- Prevention of progression of osteoporosis

Aseptic Loosening of Prosthesis

Endoprosthesis of the hip joint has become one of the most frequent and rewarding operations in orthopaedic surgery. World-wide more than 600,000 such prostheses are implanted annually. With the steady rise in life expectancy this number will also increase. Hip prostheses

Endoprostheses are stable and functional for 10-20 years, with a revision rate of only 5 % in 10 years.

last on average 10–20 years. During an observation period of 10 years there is a revision rate of 5%. In recent years the fate of these endoprostheses has been carefully followed and it appears that the biggest problem posed in the long-term is loosening of the prostheses.

Stability of the prosthesis within the bone is the decisive factor for faultless functioning. At the present technical level every endoprosthesis should be capable of full weight-bearing for 5–10 years without giving rise to any complaints. Nevertheless, *complications* increase steadily over time and the most important are:

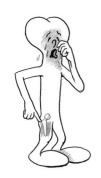

▶ Aseptic loosening
▶ Periprosthetic fractures
▶ Fracture of the diaphysis of the femur
▶ Late infections
▶ Fractures of the shaft of the prosthesis

In the long run, loosening determines the fate of the endoprosthesis. X-rays have demonstrated that the bone bordering the implant undergoes constant changes which slowly but surely lead to loosening and instability. This is the main reason for the increasing number of revision operations as the years pass. The phenomenon of loosening is now well characterised clinically, radiologically, and histologically. Three factors determine the tendency for loosening:

Eventually aseptic loosening may occur because of changes in the bone surrounding the implant.

▶ *Tissue compatibility of the implant.* The normal close approximation of osteoblasts to the implant may be hindered either by a foreign body reaction in the form of a connective tissue membrane or a foreign body granuloma – all of which trigger a periprosthetic osteolysis.
▶ *Micromovements* or friction between the two surfaces: The greater the area of friction, the more osteoclasts are activated and it is they who cause the osteolytic loosening of the prosthesis. Many biochemical mediators are involved: cytokines, prostaglandin E, metalloproteases, and collagenases. Eventually, the osteolytic regions around the shaft appear as "radiolucent lines" between bone and implant.
▶ *Release of small particles* (especially polyethylene) and formation of granulomas.

The following *factors* are decisive for the stability or the loosening of a prosthesis:

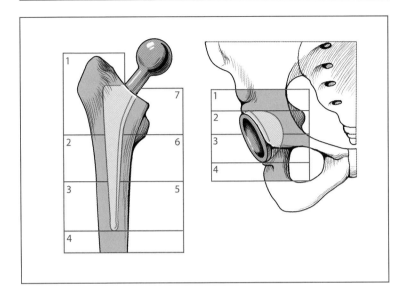

Fig. 18.7. Zones of loosening of prosthesis according to Gruen

▶ Design of the prosthesis
▶ Positioning of the prosthesis
▶ Nature of the cementing materials
▶ Method of cementing
▶ Degree of particle release and formation of foreign body granulomas
▶ Occurrence of dislocation
▶ Time since operation-insertion
▶ Local pressure on the housing of the prosthesis
▶ Structure of the adjacent bones
▶ Degree of systemic and local osseous remodelling.
▶ Degree of migration
▶ Insidious infections with nonvirulent organisms

Slight loosening remains symptomless for long periods. Extensive loosening causes considerable pain on weight bearing and on sudden sharp movements, eventually resulting in complete failure of that hip. Pain on inward rotation of the leg indicates loosening of the shaft. The X-ray findings provide evidence of the loosening. *Radiolucent lines* more than 2 mm wide indicate loosening, but localised, limited osteolyses do not constitute evidence. "Migration" of the prosthesis over

Pain on weight-bearing and on sudden movement indicate extensive loosening which eventually results in failure of that hip.

time is also diagnostic. A "migration" of >5 mm indicates loosening. A slow wandering of the cup into the pelvis frequently causes lyses in the bones and requires reimplantation. A bone scan and in certain cases arthrography may be useful, but not CT or MRI because of metallic artefacts. Bone loss in the different zones of Gruen can now be measured by DXA technique.

Causative therapy consists of replacing the prosthesis. Indications for this are pain, loosening, and migration. The accompanying osteolyses may turn this operation into a more dangerous and more difficult one than the original implantation. However, advances in technology and in materials for cementing will undoubtedly improve the long-term results. Implantation of prostheses without cement is recommended for younger patients as less bone is removed, which ensures a more favourable situation if a replacement has to be made later.

Early employment of aminobisphosphonates does not prevent loosening, but it does delay it. In cases where implantation of a prosthesis could be expected or is already planned, *preventive therapy* with bisphosphonates should be given in the following situations:

Bisphosphonates cannot absolutely prevent loosening, but may delay it.

▶ Underlying Paget's disease of bone: oral or intravenous therapy given 3–6 months beforehand will normalise the increased osseous remodelling.
▶ Underlying systemic or local osteoporosis: a steady increase in bone density for 1–3 years will enable a more stable and longer-lasting fixation of the implant.
▶ Underlying inflammatory joint disorder: inhibition of osteoclasts and suppression of prostaglandin secretion can halt the local resorption and formation of osteolytic lesions.
▶ In particular, arthrosis of the hip with its attendant erosions constitutes an important indication for preventive therapy.

After successful implantation, bisphosphonates are used to prevent loosening:

▶ Prevent osteoclastic resorption at the border interface – between implant and bone
▶ Prevent local osteolyses in vicinity of foreign body granulomas, in which the inhibition of prostaglandin secretion plays a significant part
▶ Prevent the dissolution of bone from around the prosthesis

► Delay migration, which depends on the degree and extent of re-modelling
► Inhibit heterotopic calcification and ossification
► Treat the frequently pre-existing immobilisation osteoporosis

Increases in bone mineral density improve the conditions for a later replacement operation.

More clinical trials with large numbers of patients are necessary to provide statistical evidence for these statements.

The following *treatment protocols* are recommended. Dosages and time intervals depend on the underlying condition and on the rate of bone remodelling:

► Alendronate (Fosamax)   10 mg orally daily
► Alendronate (Fosamax)   70 mg orally once weekly
► Risedronate (Actonel)   5 mg orally daily
► Risedronate (Actonel)   35 mg orally once weekly
► Pamidronate (Aredia)   30–60 mg i.v. every 3 months
► Ibandronate (Bondronat)   2–4 mg i.v. every 3 months
► Zoledronate (Zometa)   2–4 mg i.v. every 3 months

Therapy with bisphosphonates must always be combined with supplementation of 1,000 mg/d calcium and 1,000 IE/d vitamin D, especially to prevent a secondary, reactive hyperparathyroidism.

After re-implantation therapy, bisphosphonates together with calcium and vitamin D should always be given and monitored regularly by DXA measurement of the surrounding bone.

The following parameters are used to *monitor therapy*:

► Decrease in pain
► Flexibility
► X-rays over time
► DXA – bone density measurements
► Markers of bone remodelling in serum/urine
► Bone scan

The quality of bone remains unchanged even after long-term administration of bisphosphonates, which should be continued even if fractures occur, as bisphosphonates increase callus formation and lead to faster healing.

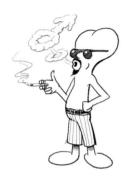

Sexual equality! Osteoporosis does not discriminate – men are as vulnerable as women. It just strikes them a few years later– and not only the trabecular network, but also the cortical bone, which further increases the fracture risk.

Clinical Evaluation in Men

Men are not immune to the progressive bone loss that occurs with ageing, with a peak 10 years later than women.

Ageing in men is accompanied by a steady decline in levels of gonadal steroids and growth hormones, which largely determine the decrease in bone mineral density. The concept of "andropause", i.e., the natural age-related decline in testosterone levels in men, is not yet widely understood by health care professionals nor the general public. It follows that there is also insufficient awareness of the benefits of testosterone replacement therapy, which has proved its value in the relatively short term while the long-term results are awaited. Moreover, so far little attention has been paid to the direct effects of gonadal steroids and their decline on bone and its metabolism in elderly men. Nevertheless, age is recognised as the most important risk factor for male osteoporosis, which occurs about 10–15 years later than that of females. That is, at about 60 years of age with an acceleration of bone loss after 70 years, apparently due to increased resorption not matched by increased formation. It should be noted that a high proportion of men (approximately 60 % in some studies) no longer have optimal secretion of androgens from 60 years of age although levels start to decrease much earlier.

The direct cause is greater resorption than formation, but decrease in muscle mass and in physical activity also contribute.

Decline in other factors associated with ageing may also contribute to osteoporosis. A decrease in muscle mass ("sarcopenia") is common even in healthy people over 60 years and increases with age and influences the status of the bones. Directed efforts to prevent the muscle loss should include sustained physical activity as the years pass and appropriate exercises.

It is only in recent years that osteoporosis in men has been recognised as a major public health problem, the extent of which is increasing steadily. For example, the cost of osteoporosis in men for the year 1999 in France was calculated according to hospitalisations caused by 21,857 fractures at a total cost of 198 million euros. In Britain, the cost has been estimated at a quarter of a billion pounds (perhaps more by now) annually. Moreover, men with hip fractures have a higher morbidity and mortality than women. This is graphically highlighted by a recent report on "Outcomes and secondary prevention strategies for male hip fractures," which draws the conclusion that men with hip fractures received inadequate evaluation and treatment for osteoporosis; however, the situation has begun to change for the better, as more data are published and public awareness increases. The first large population-based study carried out in many countries in Europe – the European Prospective Osteoporosis Study (EPOS), has confirmed the frequent occurrence of vertebral fractures in men and their increase with age. Criteria for the densitometric diagnosis of osteoporosis in men have been recommended and published.

According to recent estimates, 20 % of all cases of osteoporosis occur in men. The estimated number of men with osteoporosis in the USA is now put at 5 million (2003). Osteoporosis is present in 6 % and osteopenia in 47 % of males over age 50. The clinical picture of established osteoporosis in men is comparable to that in women, with kyphosis due to wedge fractures of the thoracic column, protuberance of the abdomen, and transverse skin folds over the dorsal trunk. The male:female ratio of hip fractures has been calculated to be 1:3 and the vertebral fracture ratio even approaches 1:2. Four *diagnostic steps* are recommended:

▶ Exclusion of other bone disorders with diminished bone mineral content (osteomalacia)
▶ Quantitation of the degree of osteopenia (DXA of lumbar spine and proximal femur, and possibly additional sites as indicated in the individual patient)
▶ Evaluation of the clinical stage of osteoporosis (preclinical – uncomplicated – advanced)
▶ Exclusion of a secondary osteoporosis (single pathogenic factor or combination of causes)

If the 47 % of men over age 50 with osteopenia were properly treated, osteoporosis and fractures would be avoided.

In young men, especially, transient osteoporosis of the hip must be distinguished from avascular necrosis, which is done by the distinctive, typical MRI findings in the former condition. Establishing the correct diagnosis avoids unnecessary surgery.

The percentage of men with secondary osteoporosis rises to 50 % – higher by 10 % than that of women. Taking this high frequency into account, the index of suspicion should also be high and men carefully screened to seek out any underlying causes for the osteoporosis.

Secondary osteoporosis occurs in 50–60 % of men and therefore the possible conditions must be carefully excluded. Three risk factors are especially relevant in men: smoking, alcohol and decreased levels of testosterone.

Important *risk factors* are:
▶ Heavy smoking
▶ Hypogonadism
▶ High alcohol consumption
▶ Hyperthyroidism
▶ Hepatic disorders
▶ Neoplasias of the bone marrow
▶ Congenital disorders of collagen metabolism

Testosterone levels must always be determined and specific causes for hypogonadism ruled out.

The most frequent cause (about 30 %) of osteoporosis in men is testosterone deficiency and it is believed to be a risk factor for hip fractures. The level of testosterone in the blood must always be determined since some patients do not suffer from sexual dysfunction and appear to have normal testes despite decreased levels of testosterone. Causes of *hypogonadism* include:

▶ Klinefelter syndrome
▶ Prolactinomas
▶ Kallmann syndrome
▶ Prader-Willi syndrome
▶ Male Turner syndrome (Noonan syndrome)
▶ Hemochromatosis
▶ Status post-orchitis
▶ Castration

Receptors for both oestrogen and testosterone are present in the male skeleton.

Testosterone deficiency in men causes an increase in resorption as well as a decrease in formation and thereby a rapid loss of bone. Moreover, it has been demonstrated in several studies that oestrogen deficiency also plays an important part in causing osteoporosis in men by the following mechanism: a high serum level of the sex hormone-binding globulin reduces the availability of both testosterone and oestrogen in peripheral tissues, including the bones. This further reduces the availability of androgen for synthesis of oestrogen by aromatisation in peripheral tissues. It is oestrogen deficiency rather than androgen deficiency which is responsible for increased bone resorption – even in men. Indeed, oestrogen action is clearly essential for normal bone development in young males, and probably exerts important effects on bone in adult men as well. Therefore, SERMs may have applications in men at risk of bone loss. A short-term trial of raloxifene in older men revealed reductions in bone markers in men with the lowest oestradiol levels. Long-term trials are needed to show the effectiveness and safety of raloxifene and in what male populations they may be most useful. An increase in serum leptin also reduces bone formation and thereby BMD. It has been postulated that the age-related difference in serum PTH levels and in bone resorption between men and women is due to more residual testosterone in men than oestrogen in women. An increase in serum leptin also reduces bone formation and thereby BMD.

> Low serum estradiol is a major risk factor for hip fracture in men.

> Advantage of oestrogen receptors on bone cells in men: could be utilised for therapy with raloxifene (SERMs), as already shown in short-term studies!

Special Features in Men

There are differences in frequency and in fracture site between men and women. Boys have fractures of the extremities more frequently than girls. However, this is readily explained by the fact that boys practice more sport than girls, particularly aggressive and contact sports, and by the stronger physical force of young men. The diameter of the vertebral bodies and of the long bones is greater in men than in women and thereby acts as an important defence against fractures. The frequency of femoral neck fractures in men decreases during the period of 35–60 years of age and only begins to rise again after 70 years. Two main factors determine the differences in the condition of the skeleton between men and women. The first is the peak bone mass and the second is the late and slow decline in testosterone. Due to their greater physical activity and higher calcium intake, young men have a peak bone mass 25% greater than that of young women. Moreover, the age-related bone loss that begins around 30 years of age is slower in men: 0.3% annually compared to 0.8% in women. Testosterone levels in men decline slowly with age so that a "male menopause" or "andropause" as it is now sometimes called, due to a sudden decrease in sexual hormones does not occur. Women may lose up to 40% of their trabe-

> Men suffer only 25% of all hip fractures, but the overall cost and resulting deaths are actually greater in men than in women.

cular bone during their lifetime but men only about 14%. The low incidence of osteoporosis in men can be explained by:

▶ A higher peak bone mass at maturity
▶ Greater diameter of the long bones and vertebral bodies
▶ A low rate of bone loss in later life
▶ Men do not undergo the equivalent of a menopause
▶ Men on average have a lower life expectancy but this is changing (fortunately)

Prevention and Treatment in Men

Testosterone replacement therapy will not help those with normal testosterone levels.

Prevention of osteoporosis in men starts with investigation of calcium intake and blood levels of testosterone, which can be given as needed by gel, patches, tablets, or i.m. injections, for example 250 mg testosterone enanthate i.m. every 3–4 weeks or testosterone patches 2.5 mg daily, though not of course to patients with carcinoma of the prostate. The following program can be applied for prevention of osteoporosis in men:

▶ Daily intake of 1,000 mg calcium and 1,000 IU vitamin D
▶ Regular physical activity, adapted to each patient
▶ No smoking
▶ Moderate alcohol consumption only
▶ Monitoring of testosterone levels and treating as required
▶ Monitoring additional disorders and medications possibly affecting the bones
▶ Avoidance of falls and use of hip protection especially in elderly men

It is reasonable to expect that the nonhormonal therapies (bisphosphonates, PTH) available for postmenopausal osteoporosis will work similarly in males.

Therapy of osteoporosis in men. The same guidelines apply as for women: adequate calcium, vitamin D, and exercise should be encouraged. If the testosterone levels are found to be low, intramuscular, subcutaneous, or transdermal testosterone will increase bone mass. As demonstrated in clinical trials, the aminobisphosphonates are equally effective, safe, and well-tolerated in men as in women and are especially indicated when sex hormone levels are within the normal range. Alendronate has been approved and is the bisphosphonate of choice for osteoporosis in men as demonstrated in prospective studies. It is worth emphasizing that a low BMD is associated with a higher risk of mortality in men and therefore adequate and early prevention is even more important.

In spite of the efficacy of antiresorptive therapy, it is clear that anabolic agents to stimulate bone formation could also play a significant part in prevention and therapy of primary osteoporosis in men. In this context, several reports have suggested that parathyroid hormone, especially as low-dose intermittent therapy, results in significant increases in BMD in male osteoporosis; however, results of long-term studies (more than 1 year) have not yet been published. Another novel treatment is short-term administration of growth hormone together with testosterone, which appeared to have a favourable effect on BMD, but long-term results of this combination are still awaited. Finally, more attention has been paid in recent years to replacement therapy in men; several options are under investigation and results should be published soon. These options include SERMs, calcitonin, and PTH alone or in various combinations. SERMs have already been used to maintain bone mineral density in men during androgen deprivation therapy. A different approach to replacement therapy recently advocated is transdermal oestrogen, which avoided or substantially reduced the unwanted side effects but proved effective at a tenth of the cost of conventional hormone therapies in men with androgen deprivation due to prostate cancer.

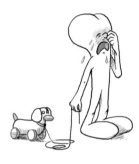

CHAPTER 20 Osteoporosis: Even More Harmful in Children

During growth, the shape, architecture, and strength of bones are modulated by three major processes: growth, modelling, and remodelling. Modelling is of particular interest as it appears that bone is much more capable of responding to external loads during growth than at any other time. Remodelling also occurs during growth, but the net result of remodelling is to lose or maintain, but not to gain bone. Information on the pattern of bone mineral accrual is illustrated in Figs. 20.1 and 20.2, which show plots and velocity curves of total body bone mineral content during growth. The authors of these longitudinal studies of boys and girls have also shown that, on average, 26% of adult total bone mineral was accrued during the 2 years around peak bone mineral content velocity, at age 12.5 for girls and 14.1 for boys. Furthermore, it is of interest that true bone density does not increase with size or age, and reported increases in BMD with age are a reflection of growth and an increase in size rather than an increase in bone mineral per unit volume.

In children, increases in bone density with age reflect growth and increase in size rather than an increase in bone mineral per unit volume.

First Clarification: Hereditary or Acquired?

Osteoporosis should be viewed as "guilty until proven innocent" of fractures in children.

Though osteoporosis rarely occurs in children, it may cause severe pain, multiple fractures, and life-long limitations of movement and locomotion when it does occur. Osteoporosis in children is often not diagnosed until after one or two fractures have occurred or if low density is suspected on X-rays. Consequently, increased awareness is just as important, if not more so, than for adults, as any decrease in bone density during childhood and adolescence which remains uncorrected will have a negative impact on peak bone mass with increased risk of later osteoporosis.

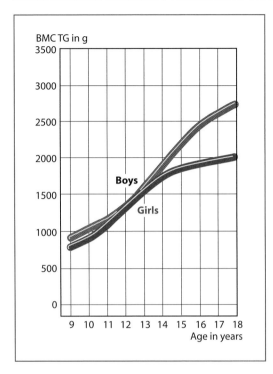

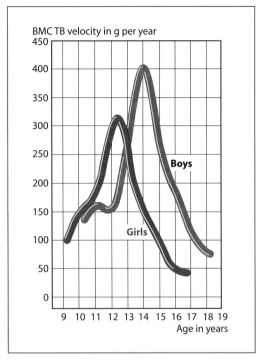

Fig. 20.1. Total body bone mineral content for boys and girls according to age. (From Bailey [A2])

Fig. 20.2. Velocity curves depicting sex and age differences in timing and magnitude of peak bone mineral accrual. (From Bailey [A2])

Osteoporosis in children has not yet been officially defined. The *WHO definition* is based on values for adults. In practice, however, the diagnosis is also based on a bone density measurement:

▶ More than 2 SD below the average value of a child of similar age with healthy bones
▶ Number of pathologic fractures

Since criteria for children have not yet been established, the parameters used for adults are applied. Cortical thickness is greater in boys than in girls at all ages.

The major causes of osteopenia/osteoporosis in children include a broad spectrum of underlying disorders, both congenital and acquired in alphabetical order (this list is not exhaustive):

Extensive investigations are required in children: blood and urine, physical and radiological examinations to rule out the numerous causes of a secondary osteoporosis.

Table 20.1. Investigation for underlying disease in childhood osteoporosis

- Complete blood count and ESR
- Renal and liver function (serum)
- Glucose (serum, urine)
- TSH (serum)
- Calcium, phosphate (serum)
- Alkaline phosphatase (serum)
- Vitamin D and PTH (serum)
- Fasting urine calcium
- X-ray skull and lumbar spine
- Bone turnover markers
- Bone/bone marrow biopsy (when indicated)

▶ Acute leukaemias
▶ Anorexia nervosa
▶ Anticonvulsant therapy
▶ Asthma bronchiale
▶ Biliary atresia
▶ Cerebral palsy
▶ Chronic hepatic disorders
▶ Chronic renal insufficiency
▶ Crohn's disease
▶ Cushing's syndrome
▶ Cyanotic congenital heart disease
▶ Cystic fibrosis
▶ Diabetes mellitus
▶ Glycogen storage disorders
▶ Growth hormone deficiency
▶ Homocystinuria
▶ Hypogonadism (e.g., Turner's and Klinefelter syndromes)
▶ Idiopathic hyperphosphatasia
▶ Juvenile chronic arthritis
▶ Malabsorption syndromes
▶ Organ transplantations
▶ Spinal cord injury
▶ Thalassemia

Acute immobilisation decreases bone formation and increases bone resorption. Additionally, bone growth is severely impaired in pro-

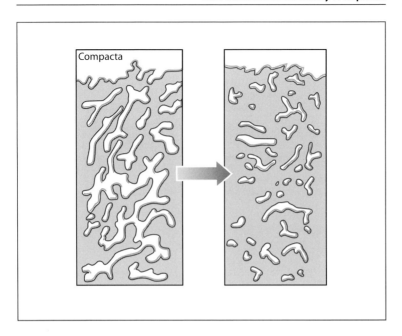

Fig. 20.3. Immobilisation os-teoporosis in a child after 17 weeks of bed rest: marked reduction in trabecular and cortical bone volume docu-mented in sequential iliac crest biopsies. (From Bartl and Frisch [B5])

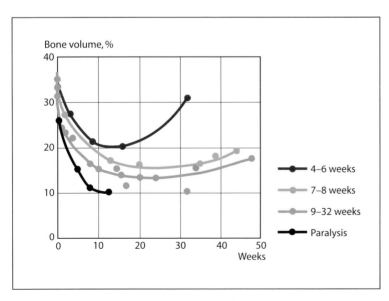

Fig. 20.4. Periods of immobi-lisation and recovery of bone mass in children. Lack of re-covery after paralysis

Bed-bound bones are in the trivial loading zone and thus rapidly lose bone mass, at a rate of about 1 % trabecular bone per week.

longed immobilisation, due to a lack of mechanical stimulation. Further important *mechanisms* of osteoporosis in children include:

▶ Inadequate production of collagen type I (congenital disorders)
▶ Prolonged immobilisation (Fractures or neurological disorders)
▶ Inflammatory cytokines (chronic rheumatic disorders)
▶ Deficiency of vitamin D (nutrition and gastrointestinal disorders)
▶ Neoplastic diseases of the bone marrow (oncological disorders)
▶ Therapy with glucocorticoids and immunosuppressive drugs.

Treatment in childhood osteoporosis includes *general measures* such as

▶ Adequate pain relief in children with vertebral fractures
▶ Orthopaedic procedures to fix fractures of the long bones
▶ Physiotherapy with rehabilitation to improve muscle strength
▶ Occupational therapy if necessary
▶ Protection of the spine
▶ Periods of bed rest in paediatric illness should be minimized

With respect to therapy, the same general principles apply as for adults. In addition: calcitriol and calcitonin have some effect, and bisphosphonates have also been tried with success.

Literature on the *medical treatment* of childhood osteoporosis is limited and still not evidence-based, but some studies have been reported and the following recommendations made:

▶ *Calcium and vitamin D* supplementation is recommended though there is little evidence of benefit in the studies available.
▶ *Calcitriol* has been investigated in several small studies with improvement in symptoms, fracture risk, and BMD, though not significantly.
▶ *Growth hormone* is a powerful anabolic agent and it is well established that children with growth hormone deficiency benefit from growth hormone therapy.
▶ *Calcitonin* is known to inhibit bone resorption and some small studies have shown that bone pain may disappear and radiographic signs of osteoporosis may improve under intranasal administration of calcitonin.
▶ *Bisphosphonates* have also been investigated in childhood osteoporosis and there have been several encouraging studies in idiopathic juvenile osteoporosis and osteogenesis imperfecta. Concern has been expressed about potential adverse effects on the growing

skeleton, though these have not appeared so far and sequential bone biopsies showed normal, lamellar bone without development of osteomalacia. There were also no adverse effects on fracture healing or growth rate. Indeed, nitrogen-containing bisphosphonates are a treatment option in childhood osteoporosis, but randomised controlled studies are required. Although not yet approved by the FDA for the use in children, nitrogen-containing bisphosphonates demonstrated benefit to the child with no serious adverse effects. Indeed, bisphosphonates are the first agents to provide the paediatrician with the opportunity to treat childhood bone disorders efficiently.

It is important to realize that *spontaneous improvement* without any medical treatment may occur. Thus, in some children with osteoporosis it may be appropriate to monitor their progress over time and "watch and wait," particularly if they appear to have stopped breaking their bones. This would also depend on the cause.

Idiopathic Juvenile Osteoporosis (IJO) and Other Conditions

In the absence of a primary causative condition, the diagnosis of *"idiopathic juvenile osteoporosis"* (IJO) is made. It is a transient, nonhereditary, rare form of childhood osteoporosis without extraskeletal involvement. In the absence of fractures, the term "osteopenia in childhood" would be more appropriate. It is important to exclude other possible causes of vertebral collapse, such as the presence of acute leukaemia.

IJO: aetiology unknown (only speculation), and spontaneous remission is the rule.

The *aetiology* of IJO has not yet been elucidated. A decrease in osteoblastic reactivity has been reported, and consequently the skeleton no longer adequately adapts to increased mechanical loads during growth. Spontaneous remissions are the rule and with onset before puberty (mostly between 8 and 12 years of age).

Differential diagnosis. Osteogenesis imperfecta (OI) is the commonest congenitally determined condition with osteoporosis which must always be carefully excluded. Osteoporosis-pseudoglioma syndrome is a very rare congenital disorder with severe osteoporosis and blindness.

Table 20.2. Differential diagnosis between idiopathic juvenile osteoporosis (IJO) and osteogenesis imperfecta (OI)

	IJO	OI
Family history	Absent	Often positive
Onset	Late childhood	Birth or soon after
Duration	1–4 years	Lifelong
Clinical findings	Abnormal gait Metaphyseal fractures Kyphosis, back pain	Abnormal dentition Blue sclerae Long bone fractures
Growth rate	Normal	Normal or decreased
Radiologic findings	Vertebral fractures "Neo-osseous osteoporosis"	Thin cortex of long bones Wormian bones in skull
Bone biopsy	Decreased bone turnover	Increased bone turnover
Connective tissue defect	No	Collagen abnormalities

The *clinical picture* presents three different manifestations:

▶ Fractures of the extremities, especially of the trabecular bones, occasionally beginning at birth (OI?). Knee and ankle pain and fractures of the lower extremities may be present.
▶ Fractures of vertebral bodies with backache, kyphosis, decrease in height and difficulties in locomotion (walking, running).
▶ Evidence of low bone density (DXA) without pathologic fractures.

Differential diagnosis of IJO first and foremost is osteogenesis imperfecta (OI).

The *diagnosis* of IJO is made by exclusion of OI and of diseases causing secondary osteoporosis. It should be emphasized that IJO is strictly a diagnosis of exclusion and that malignancies in the marrow must be considered. Diagnosis requires X-rays of the lumbar spine in two planes. When OI is suspected, X-rays of the long bones are also required to check for the characteristic metaphyseal compression fractures. The long bones are usually of normal width in IJO; the cortex might be thinned and metaphyseal fractures are common. On X-rays, the new bone formed in metaphyseal areas appears as a radiolucent band ("neo-osseous osteoporosis"). The onset of OI is usually much earlier in life; the children often have blue sclerae and abnormalities of collagen. Bone density should preferably be measured by DXA of the lumbar vertebrae and if possible a whole body measurement. For children weighing less than 30 kg a special paediatric software program is required. The modern bone marker NTX is useful for differentiating OI and IJO.

There are no known biochemical characteristics, and alterations of bone markers are nonspecific.

With the introduction of *bisphosphonates*, therapy of osteoporosis in children is now simple and effective. Several clinical trials have already provided evidence for an increase in bone density and a reduction in fracture risk in children treated with bisphosphonates. Previous fears that such therapy might interfere with growth of the long bones have not been substantiated. In addition, the osteomalacia seen under therapy with the earlier bisphosphonates are no longer observed with the newer, more potent aminobiphosphonates, which can be given orally or as infusions at 3–6-month intervals. Since randomised clinical trials in children have not yet been carried out, treatment should only be undertaken in paediatric centres, after consultation with the Ethics Committee, and signed consent by the parents or guardians. Calcium 500–1,000 mg daily and vitamin D 500–1,000 IU daily should also be given as basic therapy. Calcitriol – the active metabolite of vitamin D – could also be considered.

> If required, therapy with bisphosphonates is safe and effective.

Patients with IJO can experience a complete recovery within some years. Growth may be somewhat impaired during the active phase of the disease, but normal growth resumes thereafter. However, in some cases IJO may result in permanent disability such as kyphoscoliosis or even collapse of the rib cage. Since children undergo spontaneous remissions, especially when there is osteopenia without fractures, a policy of watch and wait is recommended to begin with.

Osteogenesis Imperfecta (OI) Must Not Be Overlooked

This congenital condition should be considered in every case of severe osteoporosis occurring in infancy and childhood. A thorough family history and physical examination are important diagnostic aids. The spine frequently shows severe changes, but fractures occur primarily in the extremities. Different mutations of the genes for collagen type I occur. When even one of the amino acids is incorrectly incorporated into the collagen molecule, a defective molecular structure may result. As a consequence, the helical structure of collagen is altered, which in turn leads to a fault in the quality of the bone (no lamellar structure

> Prenatal diagnosis of OI is possible by ultrasound at 14–18 weeks of gestation.

and susceptible for breakdown by collagenases). In addition to bone, *other organs* that incorporate collagen type I are also effected:

▶ Thin blue sclerae, rupture of sclerae, keratoconus
▶ Anomalies of the teeth which appear brown and transparent and are liable to rapid shedding
▶ Anomalies of the heart valves and of the aorta, prolapse of the mitral valve, aortic insufficiency
▶ Deafness due to damage to the stapes in the middle ear
▶ Kidney stones and hypercalciuria
▶ Hyperplastic callus formation

OI occurs in 1 of every 20,000 live births. There are approximately 15,000 patients with OI in the USA. The condition varies from apparently typical osteoporosis to severe skeletal anomalies in childhood. Four *types* of OI are distinguished:

Severity of OI varies greatly – typing I–IV is often useful.

▶ Mild form with blue sclerae (Type I)
▶ Lethal perinatal form (Type II)
▶ Progressive deforming form (Type III)
▶ Mild form without blue sclerae (Type IV)

Previous attempts at *therapy* with fluorides were unsuccessful, as were bone marrow transplants including replacement of stromal cells. Today, early administration of bisphosphonates is the therapy of choice; in severe cases by infusions every 3 months, otherwise orally. During the past 3 years we have treated 50 patients with aminobisphosphonates. All showed impressive improvements in their conditions:

▶ Increase in bone density
▶ Increase in bone quality demonstrated in sequential biopsies
▶ Decrease in symptoms especially bone pain
▶ Striking decrease in fracture rate (before therapy up to 12 fractures annually).

Bisphosphonates – a wonder-drug for children and parents with OI!

Calcium and vitamin D are taken together with the bisphosphonates to improve the mineralisation of the newly formed bone. Results of several clinical trials of bisphosphonates (pamidronate, zoledronate, neridronate) in children and adults with OI have now been published. BMD and physical activity increased markedly under treatment with bisphosphonates and the fracture rate decreased by 65%. After 4 years of treatment with pamidronate, bone mineral content, bone volume, and volumetric bone mineral density were 154%, 44%, and 65% higher, respectively, in treated than in untreated patients who were matched for age and OI type. Patients with larger deficits in bone mass at baseline had a more marked bone mass gain during therapy. It is noteworthy that long-term adverse side effects have not been reported. On the contrary, it has been claimed that, until the advent of realistic gene therapy, bisphosphonates appear to be the most efficient way of arresting the progression of OI and improving the quality of life of the patients, irrespective of the type of collagen mutation, clinical severity, and age at start of therapy.

In this connection, it is worth mentioning that there were no serious adverse effects on the foetus when bisphosphonates were given to lactating women. No bisphosphonate was detected in the breast milk collected for 48 h after the infusion of pamidronate.

Treatment of childhood osteoporotic syndromes, however, requires an *interdisciplinary approach* including orthopaedic surgeons, physiotherapists, occupational therapists, dentists, paediatricians, and psychologists for further information and support and to care for recurrent fractures. Also appropriate organisations and support groups (e. g., the Osteogenesis Imperfecta Foundation) are important for patients and their families.

All patients with OI – at any age, with any genetic defect, any degree of severity – can be given modern bisphosphonates as long as needed.

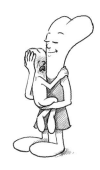

Exclusion of Secondary Osteoporoses: A Basic Necessity Before Therapy

Up to 20% of women and 60% of men presenting to specialists with osteoporosis have diseases linked to osteoporosis ("secondary osteoporosis").

The first step is the separation of "primary" or "idiopathic" from the "secondary" osteoporoses, which have an underlying cause, i.e., a specific disease or disorder. "Primary" osteoporosis refers mainly to postmenopausal and age-related involutional osteoporoses, in spite of the fact that a number of factors contributing to their pathogenesis are already known. "Secondary" osteoporoses comprise about 5% of all cases of osteoporosis but are responsible for about 20% of all osteoporotic fractures. Physicians should consider causes of secondary osteoporosis particularly among patients with:

Exclusion of secondary osteoporosis is essential in all patients at any age.

▶ Unusual fractures
▶ Very low bone densities for their age
▶ Recurrent fractures despite adherence to effective therapy
▶ Abnormal basic laboratory tests (anaemia, hypo- and hypercalcemia, elevated ESR)
▶ Unexplained bone pain
▶ Undetermined bone lesions on bone scan or X-ray (metastases, myeloma, malignant lymphomas, mastocytosis)

Osteoporosis is most likely to occur in the following disciplines. Only conditions not dealt with in other chapters are included here.

In cardiology – the main risks are decreased physical activity and anticoagulants.

Cardiology

Patients with operations of the cardiac valves and long-term anticoagulant therapy are particularly vulnerable to loss of bone. Additional

Table 21.1. Diseases and surgery associated with an increased risk of generalised osteoporosis (alphabetical list)

Diseases
Acromegaly
Addison's disease
Amyloidosis
Ankylosing spondylitis
Anorexia nervosa
Chronic obstructive pulmonary disease
Congenital porphyria
Crohn's disease
Cushing's syndrome
Diabetes mellitus
Endometriosis
Gaucher's disease
Gonadal insufficiency
Haemochromatosis
Haemophilia
Hyperparathyroidism
Hypophosphatasia
Hyperthyroidism
Idiopathic scoliosis
Immobilisation
Lactose intolerance
Lymphoma and leukaemia
Malabsorption syndrome
Mastocytosis
Metastatic disease
Multiple myeloma
Multiple sclerosis
Nutritional disorders
Osteogenesis imperfecta
Parenteral nutrition
Pernicious anaemia
Primary biliary cirrhosis
Rheumatoid arthritis
Sarcoidosis
Thalassemia
Thyrotoxicosis

Surgery
Gastrectomy
Intestinal bypass
Thyroidectomy
Transplantation

Diseases in some medical disciplines are always associated with osteoporosis. Check the list!

causes are immobilisation due to chronic cardiac insufficiency. Cardiac patients who are candidates for transplantation should also be checked for osteoporosis before and after so that fractures may be avoided.

Endocrinology

▶ Hypogonadism occurs in both sexes and has congenital-, involutional- (a normal component of the aging process), and therapy-induced forms. These forms are dealt with in the appropriate chapters in this text.

Thyroid hormones: too much or too little may cause osteoporosis!

▶ Hyperthyroidism: patients with thyrotoxicosis may have generalised osteoporosis because bone formation cannot keep up with resorption, in spite of the fact that both are increased in hyperthyroidism: a classic example of high turnover osteoporosis.

▶ Primary hyperparathyroidism (pHPT): increased secretion of parathyroid hormone due to adenomas, carcinoma, or hyperplasia produces disturbances in calcium homeostasis with release of calcium from the bones. This results in increased bone turnover and bone resorption in particular, which manifests in complex bone changes affecting both cortical and trabecular bone throughout the skeleton, and may even affect the joints. pHPT is another example of hormonally determined generalised osteopenia/porosis.

▶ Cushing's disease: This endogenous form of hypercortisolism is rare, in contrast to glucocorticosteroid-induced osteoporosis, which is common, severe, and progressive if not treated.

Osteoporosis frequently goes undiagnosed in diabetics – check for it and do a BMD!

▶ Diabetes mellitus: diabetic osteopathy occurs more frequently than is generally realised and is mainly due to inhibition of collagen production by osteoblasts. This is a direct effect of insufficient insulin secretion. An interesting observation associated with bisphosphonate therapy in type II diabetes: significant reduction in intimal thickness, suggesting an antiatherogenic effect of etidronate.

Gastroenterology

Chronic disorders of the liver or the gastrointestinal tract (e.g., malabsorption syndromes, lactose intolerance, Crohn's disease, colitis ulcerosa, pancreatic insufficiency, and primary biliary cirrhosis) frequently cause a combination of osteoporosis and osteomalacia ("osteoporomalacia") due to deficiencies of the vitamins D, K, and C. Gastric and intestinal operations (e. g., Billroth I and II and small bowel resections) interface with absorption and utilisation of calcium and vitamin D and eventually may lead to osteopathy, especially to vertebral osteoporosis. In all patients regardless of cause, administration of glucocorticoids and alcohol abuse increase the loss of bone. Large-bowel disorders are rarely associated with bone loss, since the process of absorption is generally completed in the small intestine.

Patients with gastrointestinal diseases have multiple causes for osteoporosis and osteomalacia: vigilance required!

Genetics

Studies of twins have shown that osteoporosis may be genetically determined – up to 50 % – and many genes are involved. Peak bone mass is therefore to some extent genetically programmed and the subsequent degree of loss of bone density applies especially to trabecular (cancellous) bone. Recently, the connection between the genes for vitamin D receptors and bone density have been of particular interest and subjects of research, although the results of such studies have been somewhat contradictory. Clinically, osteogenesis imperfecta is the most important of the hereditary osteoporoses. Other congenital syndromes with an osteoporotic component are: Turner, Klinefelter, Ehlers-Danlos, Marfan, and Werner. Recently, it has been shown that bone may be influenced by GH/IGFI in intrauterine (genetically determined) and postnatal life. This effect may continue into adulthood, suggesting a role for the GH/IGFI axis in the programming of bone mass in women. Results for men are awaiting publication. With successful enzyme replacement therapy in Gaucher's disease the infiltration decreases but the osteoporosis increases and should be treated prophylactically after measurement of bone mineral density. Congenital syndromes with involvement of the muscles are also prone to lead to disturbances of bone remodelling and osteoporosis.

Investigations of genetic control of skeletal development and maintenance have not yet made a practical impact. Beneficial revelations are eagerly awaited!

Haematology

Diseases of the bone marrow have a direct influence on osseous remodelling and can cause severe osteoporosis. Multiple myeloma, by way of the osteoclast-activating factors produced by the pathologic

Fig. 21.1. Osteoporotic trabecular variants: Type A in polycythemia vera and Type B in chronic myeloid leukaemia. (From Bartl and Frisch [B5])

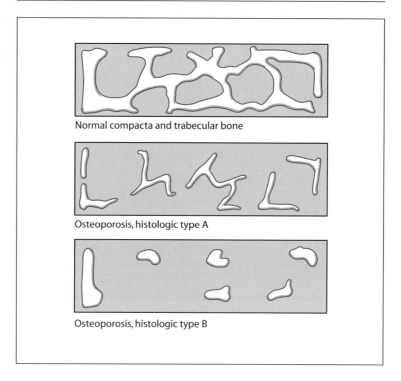

Normal compacta and trabecular bone

Osteoporosis, histologic type A

Osteoporosis, histologic type B

Bone and bone marrow are two sides of the same coin: the condition of one influences the other.

Haematopoietic, stromal and metastatic cells all secrete factors and cytokines which directly or indirectly effect bone – especially trabecular bone.

plasma cells, regularly causes osteoporosis or osteolytic skeletal lesions ("skeletal related events"). Polycythemia vera (PV) and chronic myeloid leukaemia (CML) induce widespread osteoporosis by their expansive growth, but different histological manifestations (Fig. 21.1). Similar changes are produced by congenital haemolytic conditions which cause extreme erythroid hyperplasia and osteoporosis. Storage diseases such as Gaucher's disease cause osteoporosis by comparable mechanisms. On the other hand, malignant lymphomas and acute leukaemias are rarely accompanied by osteoporosis. Systemic mastocytosis, however, is always accompanied by skeletal lesions, partly osteosclerotic, partly osteolytic, depending on the pattern of spread and topography of the mast cell granulomas. However, mast cells, because of their ability to produce and secrete heparin and histamines, probably also play a part in the pathogenesis of primary osteoporosis.

Infectious Disorders (AIDS)

In view of the fact that over 43 million people worldwide are infected with *HIV-AIDS*, this now constitutes the most important infectious disease in which osteoporosis can occur. Recent reports have shown that HIV infection is an additional risk factor for osteoporosis and pathologic fractures. Changes in bone mineral metabolism, bone histomorphometry, and bone density document the existence of a complex "AIDS-osteopathy" comprising a mixture of osteoporosis, osteomalacia, and secondary hyperparathyroidism. Immobilisation, gastrointestinal infections, lipodystrophy, hepatitis, and hormone deficiencies are all further risk factors for bone loss. Highly active antiretroviral therapy (HAART) has also been shown to accelerate bone loss in HIV-infected patients and is therefore a potent inducer of osteoporosis in these patients. The hypothesis that the systemic activation of T-lymphocytes leads to an osteoprotegerin ligand-mediated increase in active osteoclasts and bone loss may in part explain the interaction of HIV infection and bone resorption. Risk factors such as nutrition, physical activity, and other lifestyle influences also play a part in the skeletal changes listed above. With widespread introduction of treatment to delay progression of the disease, early attention should be paid to these potential complications.

> Long-term survivors in AIDS are particularly prone to osteoporosis. Therefore early detection and prevention of "AIDS osteopathy" are essential.

Nephrology

Chronic renal insufficiency induces osteoporosis, osteomalacia, and secondary hyperparathyroidism by means of deficiencies in vitamin D metabolism. During haemodialysis or after kidney transplantation, the osteopathy is somewhat improved or it may be "set" and remain static. Therapy-resistant osteoporosis is frequently encountered today as a consequence of haemodialysis. Patients with chronic renal insufficiency and long-term dialysis develop a complicated bone disorder called "renal osteodystrophy." The *manifestations* of this disorder are severe and greatly reduce the patients' quality of life: severe bone pain, multiple fractures, and extraskeletal ossifications. The extent and type of renal osteodystrophy are influenced by a broad spectrum of factors:

> Renal disorders cause a complex osteopathy, the "renal osteodystrophy".

▶ The renal disorder itself
▶ Presence of associated diseases such as diabetes mellitus and amyloidosis

▶ Severity of the renal insufficiency
▶ Patients' age – young patients are particularly severely effected, especially males up to 40 years. Subsequently, there is no differences between the sexes.
▶ Vitamin D deficiency
▶ Dietary restrictions
▶ Level of parathyroid hormones
▶ Type of dialysis and length of time patient is on dialysis
▶ Accumulation of toxic substances (e.g., aluminium, fluoride, iron)
▶ Glucocorticoid therapy

Many factors participate in the pathogenesis of renal bone disease.

Four of these factors play a decisive part in the *pathogenesis* of renal osteodystrophy:
▶ Anomalies of vitamin D metabolism
▶ Extent of secondary hyperparathyroidism
▶ Aluminium deposition on bone prevents mineralisation
▶ Immunosuppressive therapy with a negative bone balance

The metabolism of bone is also reflected in the following parameters in the *serum*: level of calcium and phosphate, bone alkaline phosphatase, intact PTH, 25- and 1,25 (OH)2 vitamin D. Aluminium and desferal tests are also useful. Levels of osteoprotegerin and PTH can also be used as indicators of high and low turnover renal osteodystrophy and reduced mineralisation in patients on haemodialysis.

Radiologic signs. These may demonstrate characteristic changes seen in osteomalacia (Looser's zones) or in secondary hyperparathyroidism such as subcutaneous and arterial calcifications, subperiosteal erosions, and "rugger jersey" spinal column.

Three components of renal osteodystrophy can be identified and classified in *histology* of bone:

▶ Alterations of remodelling: osteitis fibrosa cystica or adynamic bone
▶ Disturbance of mineralisation: osteomalacia, previously associated with aluminium
▶ Reduction in bone mass: osteopenia, osteoporosis, partly due to glucocorticoids.

A *bone biopsy* may be essential in situations in which definitive identification of the type of renal osteodystrophy is required for therapeutic decisions, as when parathyroidectomy is considered. Various histomorphometric parameters such as formation period (FP) and the quiescent period (QP) may permit a clearer identification of osteomalacia and low turnover conditions. Moreover, detailed studies of bone biopsies has led to recognition of a variant of adynamic bone disease (ABD) with PTH-independent osteoclastic resorption, which implicates other factors in osteoclast activation in these cases.

Advances in dialysis techniques and the use of active metabolites of vitamin D have radically changed the manifestations and the *therapy* of renal osteodystrophy over the last 20 years. In previous years, osteomalacia as well as secondary and tertiary HPT were major hurdles, and today severe and therapy-resistant osteoporosis is a major problem. It is characterised by markedly reduced osseous remodelling – adynamic bone disease – previously due to aluminium deposition on bone. With early institution of bisphosphonate therapy, together with active metabolites of vitamin D, the emphasis is on prevention, since early management of secondary HPT will decrease the number of patients requiring surgery. Inhibition of bone resorption in high turnover renal osteodystrophy is especially beneficial. In resistant cases with high levels of PTH and enlargement of the parathyroid glands, excision is indicated.

Three main diagnostic investigations in renal osteodystrophy are:
- Biochemistry of blood and urine
- X-ray and other imaging techniques
- Bone biopsy

Renal transplantation: important risk factor for osteoporosis!

Neurology

Chronic disorders such as Parkinson's disease, transient ischemic attacks, stroke, Alzheimer's, epilepsy, multiple sclerosis, amyotrophic lateral sclerosis, and diabetic neuropathy increase the risk of falling and correlate with lower bone mass, caused by immobility and drugs. The same is true for depressive states in which physical activity is reduced and nutrition may be inadequate. Simple and easily applicable counter-measures developed for astronauts for space flight have been advocated for patients who are paralysed to reduce bone loss. In epilepsy, some drugs such as carbamazepine used in patients, including children, also influence bone turnover so that attention must be paid to the state of the skeleton.

Osteoporosis in patients with chronic neurologic disorders is due to decreased physical activity – even immobility – drugs, and increased risk of falling.

Oncology

In patients with osteotropic tumors, metastases may cause osteoporosis or mixed osteolytic/osteosclerotic lesions. Bone pain is an early sign!

The diffuse metastatic spread of a solid tumour (usually an osteotropic one such as breast or prostatic cancer) can mimic a primary osteoporosis, particularly in the absence of osteolytic or osteosclerotic lesions. Osteoporosis of uncertain aetiology accompanied by bone pain and pathologic fractures should always be thoroughly checked to rule out an underlying malignant condition, especially of breast and prostate. The former induces mainly osteoporotic/osteolytic metastases, the latter mainly osteosclerotic. Other malignant tumours such as bronchial cancers may also cause skeletal lesions, usually paraneoplastic, by means of secretion of parathormone-related proteins (PTHrP).

Pulmonology

Chronic pulmonary diseases and their therapies are always suspects!

Patients with longstanding, cortisone-dependent asthma bronchiale should be regularly monitored for prevention of osteoporosis. Patients with cystic fibrosis may have osteoporosis even before lung transplantation and this should be treated in advance.

Rheumatology

The triad of pain, immobilisation and corticoids is characteristic of rheumatologic disorders and osteoporosis.

The combination of joint pains, immobilisation, and glucocorticoid therapy inevitably leads to a loss of bone. In patients with chronic polyarthritis, measurement of the density of the phalanges by ultrasound has proved a useful method to monitor the state of the bones.

See separate chapters for medical disciplines not included here, for example paediatrics, orthopaedics, gynaecology, surgery, and dentistry. See index for additional information in various medical disciplines.

CHAPTER 22

Osteoporosis: Many Drugs Are Bone Robbers

A detailed drug history is of vital importance, because many medicines and substances can adversely affect the skeleton. A comprehensive list of drugs associated with increased risk for osteoporosis in adults has been outlined by the National Osteoporosis Foundation.

Corticosteroid-Induced Osteoporosis

Steroid-induced osteoporosis is nearly always due to long-term therapy of one of the steroid hormones, only rarely to an endogenous Cushing syndrome. It should also be stressed that the underlying disor-

Table 22.1. Drugs associated with an increased risk of generalised osteoporosis (alphabetical list)

Aluminium antacids
Antibiotics
Anticonvulsants
Antihypertensives
Aromatase inhibitors
Chemotherapeutics
Diuretics
Glucocorticosteroids
GnRH agonists
Heparin
Immunosuppressants
Isoniazid
Lithium
Loop diuretics (e.g., Lasix)
Tamoxifen
Thyroid hormone
Warfarin

A detailed history of past and present medications is an essential component of medical investigation.

der itself often causes osteoporosis, which is then aggravated by the steroid therapy. Examples are Crohn's disease, rheumatic disorders, autoimmune disorders, organ transplants, bronchial asthma, malignant lymphomas, multiple myeloma, and others.

The use of corticosteroids over a period of days or weeks, even in very high doses, will not result in clinically significant bone loss; however, bone loss is evident within months of the start of steroid therapy. When treated over long periods of time – possibly years – about 50 % of these patients will suffer from manifest osteoporosis. Continuing bone loss is particularly likely in patients requiring more than 10 mg/day of prednisone. Children, young men, and postmenopausal women are particularly vulnerable. A few patients may have an individual sensitivity to corticosteroids. Initial bone density measurement is recommended in all patients so that a base line is established for later comparison. Corticosteroid-induced osteoporoses have the following characteristics:

> Exogenous glucocorticoid excess is the most frequent cause of secondary osteoporosis.

▶ Occur in 30 %–50 % of patients on long-term steroid therapy.
▶ Osteoporosis effects especially the trabecular bone, therefore fractures occur preferentially in vertebral bodies, ribs, and femoral neck.
▶ The rate bone loss is rapid – "fast losers," "very high turnover osteoporosis." A loss of up to 20 % of the bone mass may occur in the first year of steroid therapy.
▶ Dramatic bone loss may result from even low doses of prednisone (7.5 mg or its equivalent).

Glucocorticoids have a multifaceted *effect on bone*:

> Glucocorticoids also suppress collagen synthesis, with delayed wound healing and thinning of the skin.

▶ Inhibition of osteoblast proliferation, differentiation, and function
▶ Increased apoptosis of osteoblasts
▶ Stimulation of osteoclastic activity
▶ Decreased intestinal absorption of calcium
▶ Increased renal excretion of calcium
▶ Increased parathormone secretion
▶ Decreased secretion of calcitonin
▶ Decrease in number of bone remodelling units
▶ Occurrence of aseptic bone necroses
▶ Increased production of collagenases
▶ Decreased production of corticotropin and gonadotropin

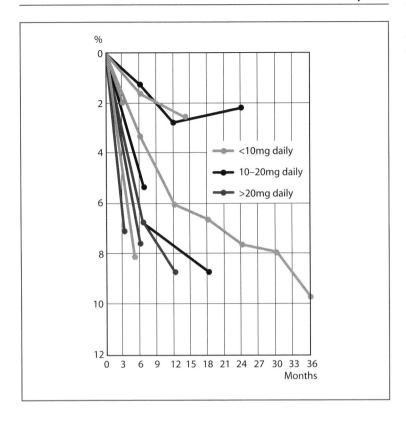

Fig. 22.1. Loss of spinal BMD from start of corticosteroid therapy. Results of ten studies. (Modified from van Staa et al [A142])

In addition, interactions of glucocorticosteroids with other factors also contribute to the pathogenesis of steroid-induced osteoporosis:

▶ Increased sensitivity of osteoblasts to PTH and to active vitamin D
▶ Decreased production of prostaglandin E
▶ Decreased local production of IGF1
▶ Effect on IGF binding proteins

Various guidelines have been developed for the therapy and prevention of corticosteroid-induced osteoporosis. The results of reviews suggest that the risk of fracture appears shortly after start of therapy and at relatively low daily doses above 5 mg/day. It is also likely that the BMD threshold for fracture is different in corticosteroid-induced osteoporosis compared to postmenopausal osteoporosis. Bone loss may

Risk of osteoporosis can be reduced by adherence to guidelines for therapy with corticosteroids.

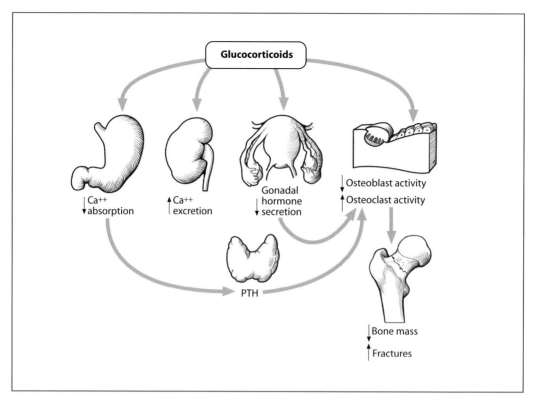

Fig. 22.2. Negative effects of glucocorticoids on calcium homeostasis, activity of bone cells and bone mass

be substantially reversible after stopping therapy and it is independent of underlying disease, age, and sex. Patients with obstructive pulmonary disease showed comparable increases in fracture risk compared to patients with arthropathies.

Even inhaled steroids may be harmful in the long term. So check their use also!

Users of *inhalation corticosteroid therapy (ICS)* also had higher risks of fracture, but this increased risk may be related to the underlying respiratory disease rather than to inhaled corticosteroid therapy. However, a quantitative systematic review has found deleterious effects of ICS on BMD. Budesonide appeared to be the ICS inducing fewer deleterious effects on bone, followed by beclomethasone dipropionate and triamcinolone.

Table 22.2. Evidence for the efficacy of interventions in glucocorticoid-induced osteoporosis

Intervention	Spine BMD	Hip BMD	Vertebral fracture	Nonvert. fracture
Calcium	–	–	–	–
Calcium + vitamin D	C	C	–	–
HRT	B	D	–	–
Testosterone	B	–	–	–
Etidronate	A	A	B	–
Alendronate	A	A	B	–
Risedronate*	A	A	A	–
Calcitriol	C	–	–	–
Alfacalcidol	A	C	–	–
Fluoride	B	–	–	–
Calcitonin	B	–	–	–

A = positive evidence from one or more large randomised controlled trials;
B = positive evidence from smaller nondefinite randomised controlled studies;
C = inconsistent results from randomised controlled studies;
D = positive results from observational studies;
– efficacy not established;
* approved for this indication

As a *general rule* one can assume that with oral therapy of more than 6 months duration at a dose of more than the equivalent of 7.5 mg prednisone/day a significant loss of bone occurs so that bisphosphonates are indicated for prevention. At higher doses, the loss of bone may rise to 15% or more per annum so that when prescribing glucocorticoids the following *recommendations* should be applied:

Use these guidelines:
- Lowest effective dose
- Shortest half-life
- Shortest duration possible
- Supportive measures

▶ Check for the lowest effective dose. Alternate day dosing does not prevent bone loss.
▶ Check for the shortest possible duration of treatment to avoid adrenal cortical atrophy.
▶ Use glucocorticoids with the shortest half-life.
▶ Utilise local application whenever possible (creams, sprays etc.).
▶ Emphasize physical activity and muscle training.
▶ Prescribe vitamin D at 1,000 IU daily.
▶ Make sure the patient consumes 1,000–1,500 mg calcium daily through diet or supplementation.

Therapy of corticosteroid-induced osteoporosis is the same as that of postmenopausal, but early use of preventive measures against corticosteroid-induced osteoporosis is highly recommended. In a recent trial, no difference was found between only vitamin D or only calcitriol, while alendronate was superior to either for treatment of glucocorticoid-induced bone loss. Therefore, the following recommendations for prevention and treatment are given:

▶ Physical activity and muscle training
▶ Calcium and vitamin D supplements
▶ Check and treat steroid-induced diabetes mellitus
▶ Check for hypogonadism and treat as needed. Administration of testosterone to men whose testosterone levels are decreased by steroid therapy may increase BMD in the lumbar spine by 5% in 12 months.
▶ Start early with a modern nitrogen-containing bisphosphonate (e.g., 70 mg alendronate once weekly or 35 mg risedronate once weekly).

Patients with intestinal absorption problems, e.g., Crohn's disease, or after a transplant are preferably treated with infusions of a nitrogen-containing bisphosphonate. Before therapy is started, bone density should be measured at the lumbar spine and the femoral neck. One of the following *treatment strategies* can then be applied according to the results:

▶ Normal bone density (T-score 2.0 to –1.0) and no additional risk factors: calcium-rich diet, vitamin D and muscle training. DXA control measurement at half yearly intervals
▶ Osteopenia and osteoporosis (T-score <–1.0): Strategy as above, plus a modern bisphosphonate orally or by infusion

Transplantation Osteoporosis

In all patients measure bone density, and start bisphosphonates – orally or intravenously – accordingly.

The number of transplants of solid organs such as kidney, liver, heart, lung, and pancreas is rising steadily together with an increase in the length of the patients' survival times. For example, 98% of kidney, 87% of hepatic, and 69% of heart transplant patients live longer than a year. Half of all transplant patients eventually develop osteoporosis with fractures and this substantially reduces their quality of life.

The *pathogenesis* of transplant osteoporosis is complex and only partly understood. General risk factors (inactivity, vitamin D deficiency, menopause, alcohol, and nicotine) and some medications (diuretics, anticoagulants, corticosteroids, and other immunosuppressive agents) are frequently involved. In addition, in many cases the diseased organ probably damaged the bone for long periods prior to transplantation. Biochemical markers of bone resorption are always elevated in the pretransplantation phase; however, the occurrence of fractures is due to immunosuppression with glucocorticoids, cyclosporin A, and tacrolimus (FK506). Azathioprine increases the number of osteoclasts but not their resorptive activity. Loss of bone is especially prominent in the first posttransplant year. Some recognized *pathogenic factors* are:

In organ transplantation, fracture incidence rates have been reported to be as high as 25–65%. Treatment and prevention strategies must target the peritransplant period, as well as the patient awaiting transplantation and the long-term transplant recipient.

▶ Prior osteopenia/osteoporosis
▶ Immunosuppressive drugs
▶ Calcium and vitamin D deficiency
▶ Hypogonadism
▶ Poor mobility
▶ Poor nutrition

Life style, nutrition, and risk factors. Previous experience has shown that years before a transplant bone density should be measured and if required the appropriate therapy should be instituted even before the transplant occurs: bisphosphonates, calcium, vitamin D or its active metabolites, and muscle training. This should prevent bone loss before transplantation. In the posttransplantation period up to 20% of the bone mass may be lost, particularly from the vertebral bodies and the femoral neck. Patients with liver, heart, and lung transplants have a particularly high rate of loss. Aminobisphosphonates and calcitriol are the first choice. Vitamin D-induced hypercalciuria must be avoided in patients with kidney transplants. In patients with hypogonadism, oestrogen or testosterone should be given. Calcium-rich diet and special exercises are also recommended for healthy bones. Calcitonin and fluoride, tested in clinical trials, were not found to be effective. Other factors such as sex and age may also impinge on osteoporosis. For example, the early rapid loss of bone in men following renal transplantation can be prevented by bisphosphonates given intravenously at transplantation and a month later.

Many factors contribute: sex, age, underlying cause, drugs, lifestyle, nutrition and physical activity. Consider all of them!

Tumour Therapy-Induced Osteoporosis

In oncology, the malignancy itself as well as the therapy may cause osteoporosis.

Many treatment protocols in oncology lead to manifest osteoporosis. Irradiation causes local atrophy of bone and bone marrow due to the toxic effects on bone cells and bone marrow, while chemo- and hormone therapy induce systemic rarefaction of both trabecular and cortical bone. Moreover, these iatrogenic effects may even be increased by a direct effect on bone of the tumour itself, which could well have preceded the deleterious effects of the therapy itself.

Chemo- and radiotherapy may be harmful to bone and may also cause nutritional problems.

Causes of osteoporosis during treatment of neoplasias are:
► Therapy-induced hypogonadism
► Glucocorticoids in chemotherapy protocols
► Toxic effects of chemotherapy
► Radiotherapy – also of the CNS in children because of brain tumours or acute leukaemias
► Immobilisation
► Nutritional disturbances

Tumour Therapy with Induction of Secondary Hypogonadism

Therapy-induced hypogonadism always causes osteoporosis, intentional in women with breast cancer and in men with prostate cancer.

Any chemotherapy with this effect will eventually also cause severe osteoporosis. Two groups of tumours are distinguished:

► Sex hormone-dependent neoplasias such as breast or prostatic cancer. Here the hypogonadism is part of the treatment strategy and substitution therapy cannot be given.
► Sex hormone-independent tumours such as Hodgkin's disease and other malignant lymphomas. In these cases, hypogonadism is an unwanted side effect.

Hypogonadism with Breast Cancer

Premenopausal patients with breast cancer develop irreversible ovarian insufficiency within the first year of chemotherapy. BMD of the lumbar spine decreases by 8%–10% and of the hips by 4%–6% within 2 years of chemotherapy. However, if bisphosphonates are given at the same time as chemotherapy, this bone loss can largely be avoided.

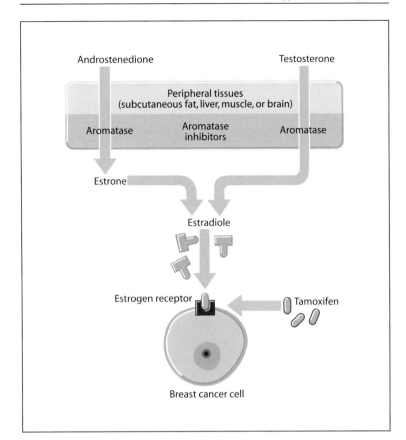

Fig. 22.3. Mechanism of action of aromatase inhibitors and tamoxifen.
(Modified from Smith and Dowsett (A129])

Moreover, therapy of ovarian insufficiency is integrated into the treatment schedule, especially of patients with oestrogen receptor positive tumours. This is achieved by means of gonadotropin-releasing-hormone (GnRH) analogues, inhibitors of aromatase (especially those of the third generation), and oestrogen antagonists. Such antihormone therapy entails a considerable long-term risk of osteoporosis. *Tamoxifen*, a synthetic antioestrogen, has an antiresorptive effect on the bone but cannot make up for the lack of oestrogen stimulation of bone formation. In contrast, *aromatase inhibitors* markedly suppress plasma oestrogen levels by inhibiting aromatase, the enzyme responsible for the synthesis of oestrogens from androgenic substrates. Unlike tamoxifen, aromatase inhibitors have no stimulatory effect on bone. Con-

In all oncologic patients osteoporosis and fractures are preventable by substitution therapy, for example SERMs or bisphosphonates.

Table 22.3. Classification of aromatase inhibitors

Generation	Type 1 (steroidal)	Type 2 (nonsteroidal)
First	None	Aminoglutethimide
Second	Formestane	Fadrozole
Third	Exemestane (Aromasin®)	Letrozole (Femara®)
		Anastrozole (Arimidex®)
		Vorozole

The steroidal aromatase inhibitor exemestane (Aromasin) also prevents bone loss in breast cancer patients with oestrogen deficiency.

sequently, nonsteroidal aromatase inhibitors of the third generation have been shown to increase the risk of osteoporosis by a profound lowering of circulating oestrogen levels. Short-term use of letrozole has been shown to be associated with an increase in bone-resorption markers, and adjuvant therapy with anastrozole is associated with a higher incidence of fractures than therapy with tamoxifen (ATAC-Study). The steroidal aromatase inhibitor exemestane, however, significantly prevents bone loss and enhances bone mechanical strength. The steroidal action of exemestane's principal metabolite 17-hydroxemestane may account for the observed bone-preserving effects.

Development of osteoporosis under nonsteroidal aromatase inhibitors or chemotherapy could be prevented or modified with concurrent use of bisphosphonates. Therefore, all patients with breast cancer should have a BMD (DXA of lumbar spine and hips) before commencing therapy. If osteopenic, *preventive therapy* with bisphosphonates should be instituted:

▶ Clodronate 1,600 mg daily per os will increase the bone mass, and most probably also decrease both skeletal and visceral metastases.
▶ Alendronate (10 mg) or risedronate (5 mg) daily orally can also be used as single therapy for prevention and treatment of osteoporosis.
▶ Alendronate (70 mg) or risedronate (35 mg) once weekly if authorised instead of the daily dose.
▶ Alternatively ibandronate 2 mg i.v. at monthly or three-monthly intervals according to the severity and activity of osteoporosis.
▶ Furthermore, zoledronate 4 mg i.v. every 6 months is also recommended and tested in clinical studies.

Patients with osteoporosis and a history of breast cancer should not receive hormone substitution therapy, but only an aminobisphosphonate orally or intravenously. Raloxifene can also be given.

Hypogonadism and Prostatic Malignancy

Attainment of hypogonadism is one of the aims of therapy, particularly in all forms of metastatic cancer and when a high postoperative PSA level is present. Possible modes of treatment are orchidectomy, GnRH analogues and antiandrogens. Patients who have received such treatments are at great risk of developing osteoporosis, and the appropriate diagnostic and therapeutic measures are indicated as for patients with mammary cancer.

Since hypogonadism is one of the major goals of therapy in patients with prostate cancer, early prevention of osteoporosis is essential to avoid fractures.

Hypogonadism in Hodgkin's Disease and Other Malignant Lymphomas

Hypogonadism resulting from therapy of the malignant lymphomas is the most frequent in the group of the nonhormone-dependent neoplasias. Irreversible ovarian insufficiency and early menopause are induced in 30%–60% of women after radio- and intensive chemotherapy. Because of the low proliferative index of Leydig cells, men are less likely to develop severe osteoporosis, though some degree of bone loss will be manifest later in life. BMD measurements should also be made in patients with lymphomas so that bisphosphonate therapy, if needed, can be given to prevent development of osteoporosis.

Drastic decreases in hormone levels occur in patients treated for lymphomas and Hodgkin's disease. Timely measurement of BMD is essential in young and older patients.

Antitumour Therapy with Direct Effect on Bone

Many protocols applied in oncology contain substances which when given systematically effect bones adversely and cause osteoporosis. However, the degree of damage and extent of bone loss depend on the frequency and/or duration of the cycles of chemotherapy. Measurement of BMD indicate when osteoporosis should be forestalled and/or treated.

Protocols Including Corticosteroids

Many protocols in oncology consist of combination chemotherapy including very high doses of glucocorticoids. Prior measurement of BMD is indicated. Short-term intermittent chemotherapy, even with high doses, does not necessarily harm the skeleton. Check anyway, it is safer!

Patients with malignant lymphomas and multiple myeloma receive chemotherapy protocols which include high doses of corticosteroids. In contrast to women with ovarian insufficiency, patients without hypogonadism did not suffer bone loss, although high cumulative doses of prednisone were given. One possible explanation may be the relatively short exposure time, in addition to which the negative impact of the bone marrow infiltration is reduced by the therapy in the lymphomas and especially in multiple myeloma.

Therapy Protocols Including Methotrexate and Doxorubicin

The effects of many therapeutic agents on the skeleton await elucidation. In the meantime take no chances – check BMD!

Many chemotherapeutic agents have not yet been investigated for their possibly harmful effects on bone. An exception is methotrexate when given for rheumatoid arthritis – increased bone resorption together with decreased formation have been reported, with an ensuing high renal excretion of calcium. One of the direct causes appears to be a drop in the recruitment of osteoblast precursors. Children treated with methotrexate (e. g., in acute lymphatic leukaemia) are especially liable to considerable resorption, although with cessation of methotrexate therapy the osteopenia is reversible. Clinical studies of bone in patients with breast cancer treated with the CMF protocol have not yet been reported.

Therapy with Ifosfamid

Changes in bone may also result from toxic effects of drugs on other organs, e.g. kidney or liver. Therefore check side effects of drugs!

This alkylating agent combined with cisplatin is used mainly for solid tumours. Depending on the amount given, it causes reversible or permanent damage of the proximal renal tubuli, resulting in metabolic acidosis, loss of phosphate, and hypercalciuria, which in turn leads to the clinical picture of osteoporomalacia. However, there is no information as yet as to whether or not ifosfamid itself has a direct toxic effect on bone cells.

Treatment Strategy

The problem of osteoporosis in patients with malignancies is underestimated. Usually, an osteologist is only consulted when the patient has already sustained one or more fractures. This unsatisfactory situation could be avoided by timely "osteoprotection," which starts with a BMD measurement when the diagnosis is established and appropriate steps taken depending on the results. These steps include the basic and specific measures outlined above.

The choice, dose, duration, and intervals of bisphosphonate therapy are determined by the severity of bone loss and the patients' risk factors. When carefully chosen and correctly administered, the bone deficit can be eradicated and a positive bone balance with increases up to 10 % in bone density obtained. A broad spectrum of bisphosphonates is available:

With increasing attention to adverse drug reactions in oncology, iatrogenic osteoporosis could be prevented in these patients. The patient's risk factors, condition and results of BMD measurement determine the choice, dose, administration, duration and intervals of antiresorptive therapy.

- ▶ Oral administration:
  - Alendronate (Fosamax)   10 mg daily
  - Alendronate (Fosamax)   70 mg once weekly
  - Risedronate (Actonel)   5 mg daily
  - Risedronate (Actonel)   35 mg once weekly
- ▶ Intravenous administration:
  - Ibandronate (Bondronat)   2 mg infusion/injection every 1–3 months
  - Pamidronate (Aredia)   30 mg infusion every 1–3 months
  - Zoledronate (Zometa)   2 mg infusion every 1–3 months
  - Clodronate (Ostac)   600 mg infusion every 1–3 months
- ▶ In summary, intravenous administration has some important advantages:
  - Supportive treatment when i.v. chemotherapy is given at 4–6 week intervals
  - Avoids gastrointestinal side effects
  - Avoids problems of gastrointestinal absorption
  - Avoids problems of compliance

Drug-Induced Osteoporomalacia

Bone formation and mineralisation require calcium and phosphate together with active metabolites of vitamin D. Drugs affecting the vita-

Osteomalacia sometimes occurs together with osteoporosis: "osteoporomalacia".

min D system may cause both osteoporosis and osteomalacia by several mechanisms:

▶ *Blockers of vitamin D production*: the elderly and institutionalised individuals with limited nutrition and sunlight exposure are at particular risk.

▶ *Inhibitors of vitamin D absorption*: vitamin D, a fat-soluble vitamin, is absorbed in the jejunum and ileum, in combination with bile acids. Therefore, bile acid-binding resins such as cholestyramine and colestipol interfere with this process and inhibit vitamin D absorption.

▶ *Interference with vitamin D metabolism*: vitamin D must be metabolised first in the liver and then in the kidney to be active. Drugs such as anticonvulsants or rifampicin induce drug-metabolising enzymes in the liver, which then accelerate the catabolism of vitamin D and its metabolites. Some reports have shown that 20%–65% of patients with epilepsy receiving anticonvulsants such as phenytoin or phenobarbital developed osteoporosis and/or osteomalacia, especially if they were institutionalised. These patients were at increased risk of fractures during their epileptic seizures. Patients taking these anticonvulsants require higher doses of vitamin D to achieve a positive calcium balance, with doses up to 4,000 IU per day. Anticonvulsants such as sodium valproate do not induce the hepatic drug-metabolising enzymes and therefore have no impact on vitamin D metabolism.

▶ *Antagonists of vitamin D action*: glucocorticoids interfere with intestinal calcium absorption, but they are not direct antagonists of vitamin D at the receptor level. There are no known drugs that directly interfere with the actions of active vitamin D at the target-tissue level.

▶ *Inhibitors of phosphate absorption*: hypophosphatemia is a major cause of osteomalacia and the most important drug-induced form is caused by excessive ingestion of aluminium-containing antacids, which inhibit intestinal phosphate absorption.

Osteomalacia has not been reported in patients on modern bisphosphonates, even long-term therapy for up to 10 years!

▶ *Inhibitors of bone mineralisation*: Aluminium-induced osteomalacia is mainly found in haemodialysis and total parenteral nutrition. Etidronate, the first bisphosphonate, also induced disturbances in mineralisation in higher doses. However, no reports of osteomalacia in osteoporosis caused by nitrogen-containing bisphosphonates have been published. Bone biopsies of patients treated with alendronate for more than 7 years have shown no evidence of demineralisation. Fluoride in higher doses often showed evidence of abnormal mineralisation, and this defect is aggravated by concomitant low calcium and vitamin D intake.

Transient Osteoporosis:
A Reaction to Local Marrow Inflammation

Transient osteoporosis of hip or joints has been ascribed to neural or circulatory mechanisms.

Transient osteoporosis may be defined as a rapidly developing painful osteopenia of benign nature and as yet unclarified aetiology. Neural and circulatory mechanisms have been considered. It is more frequent in men, though women may also be effected, especially in the third trimester of pregnancy. Spontaneous remissions occur frequently. Clinically there are 2 *groups*:

▶ Regional transient osteoporosis of the hip
▶ Regional migratory osteoporosis with involvement of various joints

Transient osteoporosis always is accompanied by local bone marrow oedema in MRI!

The patients complain of severe pain and limitation of movement in the effected joints. In the later stages, X-rays show local bone loss. MRI is needed to demonstrate bone marrow oedema near the effected joints. Occasionally, bone marrow atrophy may presage an *osteonecrosis* which can later be demonstrated by MRI. In the differential diagnosis, a localised immobilisation osteoporosis and Sudeck's disease must be ruled out.

Spontaneous remissions are frequent, but bisphosphonates can help early!

An important therapeutic measure is to relieve the joint of any stress and weight-bearing. Frequently, this is followed by spontaneous regression of the symptoms, which would seem to indicate an overloading of the joint. *Bisphosphonates* given intravenously for 4–6 months according to the following schedule are recommended:

▶ Ibandronate (Bondronat) 4 mg infusion monthly
▶ Pamidronat (Aredia) 60 mg infusion monthly
▶ Zoledronate (Zometa) 4 mg infusion monthly

Complex Regional Pain Syndrome (CRPS): Reaction to Local Neurostimulation

This syndrome is also known as algodystrophy, sympathetic reflex dystrophy (SRD), or Morbus Sudeck. This disorder still presents many unanswered questions both with respect to aetiology and to treatment. There are apparently many causes, among which are disturbances of the vegetative nervous system in the effected areas. Endocrine and psychosomatic disturbances have also been blamed. CRPS may be triggered by various factors such as fractures, operations, infections, and damage to nerves. The severity of the underlying cause appears to bear no relationship to the degree of CRPS. Most commonly involved are the hand, ankle, and knee joints. The *clinical findings* are determined by the triad of sympathetic, motor, and sensory manifestations which give rise to five main symptoms:

This syndrome appears to have many different causes; to be switched on by many different triggers; and to vary with respect to site, severity and physical manifestations. Local bone loss is typical.

▶ Strong pain
▶ Swelling and warmth
▶ Pigmentation of the skin
▶ Increased hair growth
▶ Stiffening of the joints concerned

The patients' pain and suffering are the salient clinical features of CRPS.

The *diagnosis* is established by:
▶ Thermography (area of overheating)
▶ Bone scan (area of increased uptake)
▶ X-rays (patch rarefaction of bone)
▶ MRI in early or unclear cases (oedematous areas around the joints)
▶ Alleviation of pain by blockage of the sympathetic nerve supply [designated as "sympathetically maintained pain" (SMP)]

This disorder has a chronic course and can be practically divided into *three stages*:

CRPS runs a chronic course of up to 12 months in 3 stages.

▶ *Inflammatory stage* (0–3 months): This stage is characterised by bluish discoloration and hyperthermia of the skin, together with dough-like edema and restricted movements of the joints. X-ray findings are within normal limits, but bone marrow oedema shows up on MRI.
▶ *Dystrophic stage* (3–6 months): The swelling and the hyperthermia regress and trophic skin condition develops. The movement limitations of the joint increase. The X-ray film now demon-

strates clearly a focal or a diffuse osteopenia in the effected skeletal region.

▶ *Atrophic stage* (6–12 months): This is the end stage, which is characterised by atrophy of skin, muscle, and bone. The stiffening of the joint gets worse, and there is massive focal rarefaction of the bone.

Therapy of CRPS is first and foremost symptomatic and supportive!

Attempts to *treat* the condition are frustrating as the patient continues to suffer. First, it is essential to break the vicious circle of pain and dystrophy by rest and physiotherapy. In stage I analgesics, antiphlogistic agents and stimulators of blood flow are tried. An early blockade of the stellar plexus may have a beneficial effect. In stage II and III, physical therapy and exercises should be undertaken. Surgery is only indicated for stabilisation of a fracture or later for correction of a deformity. However, it should be noted that early surgical intervention carries the risk of aggravating the condition.

Unless unavoidable, surgery is contraindicated as it may aggravate the condition.

So far, only therapy with bisphosphonates has proved successful in alleviating the pain – and, in many patients, has cured the condition!

Bisphosphonates inhibit secretion of prostaglandin E by neuromodulators so that it does not reach the nerve endings. Therefore, bisphosphonates have also been tried in inflammatory conditions of the bone and bone marrow. The first impressive positive results were obtained in patients with transitory osteoporosis. Prostaglandin E also contribute to the pathogenesis of the pain in CRPS, therefore it seemed logical to undertake trials with bisphosphonates in this condition also. Such trials have been underway since 1988 using pamidronate intravenously. All showed a decrease in pain and many patients were cured. Additional clinical trials with clodronate and alendronate have also proved to be successful. We have obtained excellent results in patients treated since 1998 with one of the following *nitrogen-containing bisphosphonates* for 4–6 months:

▶ Pamidronate (Aredia)   Infusion of 60 mg monthly
▶ Ibandronate (Bondronat)   Infusion of 4 mg monthly
▶ Zoledronate (Zometa)   Infusion of 4 mg monthly

Intravenous infusions appeared to have been particularly appropriate in these patients.

Occasionally, acute-phase reactions have occurred the day after the first infusion. Many patients – some already morphine-dependent – have been cured by this therapy. In others, the pain was alleviated to such a degree that analgesics were no longer required, and we continued with alendronate (Fosamax once weekly 70 mg). Since the bisphosphonates have nor yet been authorised for treatment of Sudeck's disease, the patients' informed consent to treatment must be obtained and documented.

Gorham-Stout Syndrome: The Ultimate Osteoporosis

Gorham-Stout syndrome is also called massive osteolysis, disappearing bone disease, vanishing bone disease, or phantom bone. This disorder was first described by Jackson in 1938 as "a boneless arm." In 1953, Gorham and Stout published 24 cases and emphasized the angiogenic component of the disease. A review of the recent literature, based on 46 patients, revealed the following *clinical features*:

▶ It affects young adults, without preference for male or female.
▶ Genetic, endocrinologic, and metabolic disturbances were not found.
▶ It starts in a single bone and proceeds to involve the adjacent bones.
▶ However, in 38 of 46 cases the condition was already polyostotic at diagnosis.
▶ Pelvis, vertebrae, ribs, proximal bones of the extremities, and skull were frequently effected.
▶ Progression and spread of the disease are unpredictable.
▶ When the ribs are effected, pulmonary insufficiency is frequently a lethal complication.

Aetiology and pathophysiology. The cause has not yet been elucidated. Haemangiomatosis and lymphangiomatosis have been implicated, possibly due to an endothelial defect, with production of abnormal high levels of cytokines that stimulate osteoclasts. Many investigators have described predominant osteoclasts, particularly in the lytic front of the lesions. However, no reactive osteoblastic activity has ever been documented showing that the physiologic "coupling" between bone resorption and formation has been abrogated. This clearly indicates a communication defect resulting in lack of stimulation and/or inhibition of osteoblasts. In one patient, Interleukin 6 (IL6, a cytokine that stimulates osteoclasts and possibly is produced by the endothelial cells) was implicated. Initially high levels of IL6 dropped after therapy with bisphosphonates and radiation.

What initiates and sustains the osteoclastic resorption in this syndrome, and how, is still a mystery. No putative causes have been discovered.

The *diagnosis* is established by X-rays which demonstrate the absence of bone in the effected areas. Occasionally, vertebral compression fractures in severe osteoporosis must be considered in the differential diagnosis. Bone biopsies taken from an involved area show increased osteoclastic resorption by morphologically normal osteoclasts. The resorption lacunae were filled with fibroblasts, blood ves-

The coupling of osteoclastic resorption and osteoblastic formation is completely abrogated.

There was no effective therapy before the advent of bisphosphonates. Osteoclastic resorption is stopped immediately by intravenous bisphosphonates.

sels, and oedematous connective tissue. Infiltration of the involved areas by plasma cells, lymphocytes, and mast cells suggests an immunological event.

Before the introduction of bisphosphonates, the disease followed an inexorable progression. All attempts at therapeutic intervention failed. Focal osteolysis can be abrogated immediately by *intravenous bisphosphonates*, which stops progression of the disease. We recommend ibandronate 4 mg infusion monthly for 4–6 months. X-rays should be taken every 4–6 months for follow-up. Restitution of the vanished bone has not been observed even under therapy with bisphosphonates.

Bibliography

Introduction

The most relevant and useful books and articles are given at the end of the text. The 28 books listed contain comprehensive summaries and reviews of the different aspects of osteoporosis published during the past 10 years or so. They also contain extensive and exhaustive reference lists.

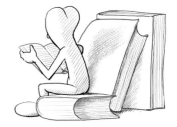

In addition to the other books recently published (not listed here), an astronomical number of articles on all aspects of osteoporosis has appeared in the international literature. These are readily available through the internet. For example, the two key words "osteoporosis therapy" yielded over 1,000 citations for the period "January to July 2003" alone. Consequently, it is clearly impossible to cite all or even most of the very recent and up-to-date articles; therefore, only a few could be listed. An attempt has been made to include articles which made specific points appearing in the text.

Books on Osteoporosis

B1. Avioli L (2000) The osteoporotic syndrome. Academic Press, San Diego
B2. Avioli L, Krane S (1997): Metabolic bone disease and clinically related disorders. Academic Press, San Diego
B3. Barlow D, Francis R, Miles A (2001) The effective management of osteoporosis. Aesculapius Medical Press, London, San Francisco, Sydney
B4. Bartl R (2001) Osteoporose – Prävention, Diagnostik, Therapie. Thieme, Stuttgart, New York
B5. Bartl R, Frisch B (1993) Biopsy of bone in internal medicine – an atlas and sourcebook. Kluwer Academic Publishers, Dordrecht, Boston, London
B6. Bartl R, Frisch B (2002) Bisphosphonates for bones: guidelines for treatment in all medical disciplines. Blackwell, Berlin
B7. Bilezikian J, Raisz L, Rodan G (1996): Principles of bone biology. Academic Press, San Diego

B8. Cummings S, Cosman F, Jamal S (2002) Osteoporosis: an evidence-based guide to prevention and therapy. American College of Physicians, Philadelphia

B9. Eastell R, Baumann M, Hoyle N, Wieczorek L (eds) (2001): Bone markers, biochemical and clinical perspectives. Martin Dunitz, London

B10. Favus MJ (ed) (1999): Primer on the metabolic bone diseases and disorders of mineral metabolism. Lippincott, Philadelphia

B11. Fleisch H (2000): Bisphosphonates in bone disease. 4th ed, Academic Press, San Diego

B12. Frisch B, Bartl R (1998): Biopsy interpretation of bone and bone marrow. Arnold, London

B13. Geusens P (ed) (1998): Osteoporosis in clinical practice. Springer, Heidelberg

B14. Henderson JE, Goltzman D (eds) (2000): The osteoporosis primer. Cambridge University Press, Cambridge

B15. Hosking D, Ringe J (2000) Treatment of metabolic bone disease – management strategy and drug therapy. Martin Dunitz, London

B16. Kanis J, Black D, Cooper C, et al. (2002) A new approach to the development of assessment guidelines for osteoporosis. Osteoporos Int 13:527–536

B17. Kleerekoper M, Siris E, McClung M (eds) (1999): The bone and mineral manual. Academic Press, London

B18. Marcus R, Feldman D, Kelsey J (eds) (1996): Osteoporosis. Academic Press, San Diego

B19. Martin B, Burr D, Sharkey N (eds) (1998) Skeletal tissue mechanics. Springer, New York

B20. Meunier PJ (1998): Osteoporosis: diagnosis and management. Martin Dunitz, London

B21. McIlwain H, Bruce D (1999) The osteoporosis cure. Avon Books, New York

B22. Mundy G (1999): Bone remodelling and its disorders. 2nd ed, Martin Dunitz, London

B23. Notelovitz M (1999): Osteoporosis: prevention, diagnosis and management. Professional Communications, Caddo

B24. Orwoll E (ed) (1999): Osteoporosis in men. Academic Press, San Diego

B25. Ringe J, Meunier P (1996) Osteoporotic fractures in the elderly. Thieme, Stuttgart

B26. Rosen C, Glowacki J, Bilzikian J (eds) (1999): The aging skeleton. Academic Press, San Diego

B27. Rubens R, Mundy G (eds) (2000): Cancer and the skeleton. Martin Dunitz, London

B28. Woolf A (1994) Osteoporosis. Martin Dunitz, London

Selected Articles in Journals

A1. Ammann P, Rizzoli R (2003) Bone strength and its determinants. 14 (Suppl3): S13–S18

A2. Bailey D (1997) The Saskatchewan pedriatic bone mineral accrual study: bone mineral acquisition during the growing years. Int J Sports Med 18 (Suppl3): 191–194

A3. Banse X (2002) When density fails to predict bone strength. Acta Orthop Scand 73, Suppl 303:S2–S53

A4. Barrett-Connor J, Grady D, Sashegyi A, et al. (2002) Raloxifene and cardiovascular events in osteoporotic postmenopausal women. Four-year results from the MORE (Multiple Outcomes of Raloxifene Evaluation) randomized trial. JAMA 287:847–857

A5. Bauer D (2003) HMG CoA reductase inhibitors and the skeleton: a comprehensive review. Osteoporos Int 14:273–282

A6. Baur A, Stäbler A, Arbogast S, et al. (2002) Acute osteoporotic and neoplastic vertebral compression fractures: fluid sign at MR imaging. Radiology 225:730–735

A7. Bilezikian J, Raisz L, Rodan G (1996): Principles of bone biology. Academic Press, San Diego

A8. Biolo G, Heer M, Narici M, Strollo F (2003) Microgravity as a model of ageing. Curr Opin Clin Nutr Metab Care 6:3–7

A9. Black D, Cummings S, Karpf D, et al. (1996) Randomised trial of effect of alendronate on risk of fracture in women with existing vertebral fractures. Lancet 348:1535–1541

A10. Black D, Thompson D, Bauer D, et al. (2000) Fracture risk reduction with alendronate in women with osteoporosis: The Fracture Intervention Trial. J Clin Endocrinol Metab 85:4118–4124

A11. Boivin G, Meunier P (2003) The mineralisation of bone tissue: a forgotten dimension in osteoporosis research. Osteoporos Int 14(Suppl3):S19–S24)

A12. Bone H, Adami S, Rizzoli R, et al. (2000) Weekly administration of alendronate: rationale and plan for clinical assessment. Clin Ther 22:15–28

A13. Bonner F Jr, Sinaki M, Grabois M, et al. (2003) Health professional's guide to rehabilitation of the patient with osteoporosis. Osteoporos Int 14 (Suppl2): S1–S22

A14. Borah B, Dufresne T, Chmielewski P, et al. (2002) Risedronate preserves trabecular architecture and increases bone strength in vertebra of ovariectomized minipigs as measured by three-dimensional microcomputed tomography. J Bone Miner Res 17:1139–1147

A15. Borderi M, Farneti B, Tampellini L, et al. (2002) HIV-1, HAART and bone metabolism. New Microbiol 25:375–384

A16. Boyle W, Simonet W, Lacey D (2003) Osteoclast differentiation and activation. Nature 423:337–341

A17. Brody B, Dickey N, Ellenberg S, et al. (2003) Is the use of placebo controls ethically permissible in clinical trials of agents intended to reduce fractures in osteoporosis? J Bone Miner Res 18:1105–1109

A18. Brumsen C, Hamdyy N, Papapoulos S (1997) Long-term effects of bisphosphonates on the growing skeleton. Studies of young patients with severe osteoporosis. Medicine 76:266–283

A19. Brumsen C, Papapoulos S, Lentjes E, et al. (2002) A potential role for the mast cell in the pathogenesis of idiopathic osteoporosis in men. Bone 31:556–561

A20. Burr D (2002) The contribution of the organic matrix to bone's material properties. Bone 31:8–11

A21. Cauley J, Norton L, Lippman M, et al. (2001) Continued breast cancer risk reduction in postmenopausal women treated with raloxifene: 4-year results from the MORE trial. Breast Cancer Res Treat 65:125–134

A22. Chapurlat R, Bauer D, Nevitt M, et al. (2003) Incidence and risk factors for a second hip fracture in elderly women. The study of osteoporotic fractures. Osteoporos Int 14:130–136

A23. Chapuy M, Arlot M, Duboeuf F, et al. (1992) Vitamin D3 and calcium to prevent hip fractures in elderly women. N Engl J Med 327:1637–1642

A24. Charles P (1992) Calcium absorption and calcium bioavailability. J Intern Med 231:161–168

A25. Chavassieux P, Arlot M, Reda C, Wei L, Yates A, Meunier P (1997) Histomorphometric assessment of the long-term effects of alendronate on bone quality and remodeling in patients with osteoporosis. J Clin Invest 1000:1475–1480

A26. Chesnut C, McClung M, Ensrud K, et al. (1995) Alendronate treatment of the postmenopausal osteoporotic women: effect of multiple dosages on bone mass and bone remodeling. Am J Med 99:144–152

A27. Chesnut C, Silverman S, Andriano K, et al. (2000) A randomized trial of nasal spray salmon calcitonin in postmenopausal women with established osteoporosis: the prevent recurrence of osteoporotic fractures study. Am J Med 109:267–276

A28. Cornell C (1990) Management of fractures in patients with osteoporosis. Orthop Clin North Am 21:121–141

A29. Cranney A, Guyatt G, Griffith L, et al. (2002) IX: Summary of meta-analyses of therapies for postmenopausal osteoporosis. Endocr Rev 23:570–578

A30. Cummings S, Black D, Rubin S (1989) Lifetime risks of hip, Colles' or vertebral fracture and coronary heart disease among white postmenopausal women. Arch Intern Med 149:2445–2449

A31. Cummings S, Black D Thompson D, et al. (1998) Effect of alendronate on risk of fracture in women with low bone density but without vertebral fractures. JAMA 280:2077–2082

A32. Currey J (2003) Perspective: how well are bones designed to resist fracture. J Bone Miner Res 18:591–598

A33. Dawson-Hughes B, Harris S, Krall E, Dallal G (1997) Effect of calcium and vitamin D supplementation on bone density in men and women 65 years of age or older. N Engl J Med 337:1437–1443

A34. Dempster D (2002) The impact of bone turnover and bone-active agents on bone quality: focus on the hip. Osteoporos Int 13:349–352

A35. Dempster D, Cosman F, Kurland E, et al. (2001) Effects of daily treatment with parathyroid hormone on bone microarchitecture and turnover in patients with osteoporosis: a paired biopsy study. J Bone Miner Res 16:1846–1853

A36. Donahue H (2000) Gap junctions and biophysical regulation of bone cell differentiation. Bone 26:417–422

A37. Einhorn T, Bonnarens F, Burstein A (1986): The contributions of dietary protein and mineral to the healing of experimental fractures: a biomechanical study. J Bone Joint Surg Am 68:1389–1395

A38. El-Shinnawi U, El-Tantawy S (2003) The effect of alendronate sodium on alveolar bone loss in periodontitis (clinical trial). J Int Acad Periodontol 5:5–10

A39. Emkey R, Delmas P, Goemaere S, et al. (2003) Changes in bone mineral density following discontinuation of alendronate therapy of glucocorticoid-treated patients: a retrospective, observational study. Arthritis Rheum 48:1102–1108

A40. Ettinger B, Black D, Mitlak B, et al. (1999) Reduction of vertebral fracture risk in postmenopausal women with osteoporosis treated with raloxifene. Results from a 3-year randomised clinical trial. JAMA 282:637–645

A41. Fleisch H (2001) Can bisphosphonates be given to patients with fractures? J Bone Miner Res 16:437–440

A42. Flier J (2002) Is brain sympathetic to bone? Nature 420:619–622

A43. Follin S, Black J, McDermott M (2003) Lack of diagnosis and treatment of osteoporosis in men and women after hip fracture. Pharmacotherapy 23:190–198

A44. Freedman K, Kaplan F, Bilker W, et al. (2000) Treatment of osteoporosis: are physicians missing an opportunity? J Bone Joint Surgery 82:1063–1070

A45. Gardner M, Flik K, Mooar P, et al. (2002) Improvement in the undertreatment of osteoporosis following hip fracture. J Bone Joint Surgery 84:1342–1348

A46. Garfin S, Yuan H, Reiley M (2001) New technologies in spine: kyphoplasty and vertebroplasty for the treatment of painful osteoporotic compression fractures. Spine 26:1511–1515

A47. Gerdhem P, Obrant K (2002) Effects of cigarette-smoking on bone mass as assessed by dual-energy X-ray absorptiometry and ultrasound. Osteoporos Int 13:933–936

A48. Gerdhem P, Akesson K, Obrant K (2003) Effect of previous and present physical activity on bone mass in elderly women. Osteoporos Int 14:208–212

A49. Glorieux F, Bishop N, Plotkin H, et al. (1998) Cyclical administration of pamidronate in children with severe osteogenesis imperfecta. N Engl J Med 339:947–952

A50. Goodship A, Lawes T, Green J., et al. (1999) Bisphosphonates can inhibit mechanically related loosening of hip prostheses. J Bone Joint Surg (Br) 81-B: Supp III

A51. Grados F, Depriester C, Cayrolle G, et al. (2000) Long-term observations of vertebral osteoporotic fractures treated by percutaneous vertebroplasty. Rheumatology 39:1410–1414

A52. Grady D (2003) Postmenopausal hormones – therapy for symptoms only. N Engl J Med 348:1835–1837

A53. Gregg E, Pereira M, Caspersen C (2000) Physical activity, falls, and fractures among older adults: a review of the epidemiologic evidence. J Am Geriatr Soc 48:883–893

A54. Grisso J, Kelsey J, Strom B, et al. (1991) Risk factors for falls as a cause of hip fracture in women. N Engl J Med 324:1326–1331

A55. Gruen T, McNeice G, Amstutz H (1979) "Modes of failure" of cemented stem-type femoral components: a radiographic analysis of loosening. Clin Orthop 141:17–27

A56. Gueldner S, Burke S, Smiciklas-Wright H (2000) Preventing and managing osteoporosis. Springer Publishing Company, New York

A57. Hornby SB, Evans G, Hornby SL, et al. (2003) Long-term zoledronic acid treatment increases bone structure and mechanical strength of long bones of ovarectomized adult rats. Calcif Tissue Int 72:519–527

A58. Häuselmann H, Rizzoli R (2003) A comprehensive review of treatments for postmenopausal osteoporosis. Osteoporos Int 14:2–12

A59. Haguenauer D, Welch V, Shea B, et al. (2000) Fluoride for the treatment of postmenopausal osteoporotic fractures: a meta-analysis. Osteoporos Int 11: 727–738

A60. Harper K, Weber T (1998) Secondary osteoporosis. Diagnostic considerations. Endocrinol Metab Clin North Am 27:325–348

A61. Harada S, Rodan G (2003) Control of osteoblast function and regulation of bone mass. Nature 423:349–355

A62. Harris S, Watts N, Genant G, et al. (1999) Effects of risedronate treatment on vertebral and nonvertebral fractures in women with postmenopausal osteoporosis. JAMA 282:1344–1352

A63. Hartman C, Hochberg Z, Shamir R (2003) Osteoporosis in pediatrics. Isr Med Assoc J 5:509–515

A64. Heinemann D (2000) Osteoporosis. An overview of the National Osteoporosis Foundation clinical practice guide. Geriatrics 55:31–36

A65. Hochberg M, Greenspan S, Wasnich R, et al. (2002) Changes in bone density and turnover explain the reduction in incidence of nonvertebral fractures that occur during treatment with antiresorptive agents. J Clin Endocrinol Metab 87:1586–1592

A66. Hofman S (1999): Bone marrow oedema in transient osteoporosis, reflex sympathetic dystrophy and osteonecrosis. EFORT 4:138–151

A67. Hollon M, Larson E, Koepsell T, Downer A (2003) Direct-to-consumer marketing of osteoporosis drugs and bone densitometry. Ann Pharmacother 37:976–981

A68. Hosking D, Chilvers C, Christiansen C, et al. Prevention of bone loss with alendronate in postmenopausal women under 60 years of age. N Engl J Med 338:485–492

A69. Hughes-Fulford M, Tjandrawinata R, Fitzgerald J, et al. (1998) Effects of microgravity on osteoblast growth. Gravit Space Biol Bull 11:51–60

A70. Johnell O, Kannus P, Obrant K, et al. (2001) Management of the patient after an osteoporotic fracture: guidelines for orthopedic surgeons. Acta Orthop Scand 72:325–330

A71. Johnell O, Oden A, De Laet C, et al. (2002) Biochemical markers and the assessment of fracture probability. Osteoporos Int 13:523–526

A72. Kanis J, Black D, Cooper C, et al. (2002) A new approach to the development of assessment guidelines for osteoporosis. Osteoporos Int 13:527–536

A73. Juby A, De Geus-Wenceslau C (2002) Evaluation of osteoporosis treatment in seniors after hip fracture. Osteoporos Int 13:205–210

A74. Kamel H, Hussain M, Tariq S, et al. (2000) Failure to diagnose and treat osteoporosis in elderly patients hospitalized with hip fracture. Amer J Med 109: 326–328

A75. Kannus P, Parkkari J, Niemi s, et al. (2000) Prevention of hip fracture in elderly people with use of a hip protector. N Engl J Med 343:1506–1513

A76. Katzman D (2003) Osteoporosis in anorexia nervosa: a brittle future? Curr Drug Target CNS Neurol Disord 2:11–15

A77. Key L, Ries W, Madyastha P, Reed F (2003) Juvenile osteoporosis: recognizing the risk. J Pediatr Endocrinol Metab 16(Suppl3):683–686

A78. Klift M, Laet C, Coebergh J, et al. (2003) Bone mineral density and the risk of breast cancer: the Rotterdam study. Bone 32:211–216

A79. Kudlacek S, Freudenthaler O, Weissboeck H, et al. (2003) Lactose intolerance: a risk factor for reduced bone mineral density and vertebral fractures? J Gastroenterol 37:1014–1019

A80. Levy P, Levy E, Audran M, et al. (2002) The cost of osteoporosis in men: the French situation. Bone 30:631–636

A81. Liberman U, Weiss S, Bröll J, et al. for the Alendronate Phase III Osteoporois Treatment Study Group(1995) Effect of oral alendronate on bone mineral density and the incidence of fractures in postmenopausal osteoporosis. N Engl J Med 333:1437–1443

A82. Lieberman I, Dudeney S, Reinhardt M-K, et al. Initial outcome and efficacy of "kyphoplasty" in the treatment of painful osteoporotic vertebral compression fractures. Spine 26:1631–1638

A83. Lippuner K, von Overbeck J, Perrelet R, et al. (1997) Incidence and direct medical costs of hospitalisations due to osteoporotic fractures in Switzerland. Osteoporosis Int 7:414–425

A84. Lips P, Graafmans W, Ooms M, et al. (1996) Vitamin D supplementation and fracture incidence in elderly persons. A randomized placebo-controlled trial. Ann Intern. Med. 124:400–406

A85. Lips P (2001) Vitamin D deficiency and secondary hyperparathyroidism in the elderly: consequences for bone loss and fractures and therapeutic implications. Endocr Rev 22:477–501

A86. Manolagas S (2000) Birth and death of bone cells: Basic regulatory mechanisms and implications for the pathogenensis and treatment of osteoporosis. Endocr Rev 21:115–137

A87. Marcus R, Wong M, Heath H, et al. (2002) Antiresorptive treatment of postmenopausal osteoporosis: comparison of study designs and outcomes in large clinical trials with fracture as an endpoint. Endocr Rev 23:16–37

A88. Maricic M, Aachi J, Meunier P, et al. (2000) Raloxifene 60 mg/day has effects within 12 months in postmenopausal osteoporosis treatment and prevention studies. Arthritis Rheum 43(9Suppl):197–201

A89. Marie P (2003) Optimizing bone metabolism in osteoporosis: insight into the pharmacologic profile of strontium ranelate. Osteoporos Int 14(Suppl 3):S9-S12

A90. Marshall D, Johnell O, Wedel H, et al. (1996) Meta-analysis of how well measures of bone mineral density predict occurrence of osteoporotic fractures. Br Med J 312:1254–1259

A91. Masud T, Mulcahy B, Thompson AV, et al. (1998) Effects of cyclical etidronate combined with calcitrol versus cyclical etidronate alone on spine and femoral neck bone mineral density in postmenopausal osteoporotic women. Ann Rheum Dis 57:346–349

A92. Mattson J, Cerutis D, Parrish L (2002) Osteoporosis: a review and its dental implication. Compend Contin Educ Dent 23:1001–1004

A93. McClung M, Eastell R, Benhamouu L, et al. (2001) Risedronate reduces hip fractures in elderly postmenopausal women. N Engl J Med 344:333–340

A94. Melton L, Heaney R (2003) Osteoporosis: too much medicine? Or too little? Bone 32:327–331

A95. Migliaccio S, Anderson J (2003) Isoflavones and skeletal health: are these molecules ready for clinical application? Osteoporos Int 14:361–368

A96. Mosca L, Barrett-Connor E, Wenger N, et al. (2001) Design and methods of the Raloxifene Use for The Heart (RUTH) study. Am J Cardiol 88:392–395

A97. Nakashima A, Yorioka N, Tanji C, et al. (2003) Bone mineral density may be related to atherosclerosis in hemodialysis patients. Osteoporos Int 14:369–373

A98. Neer R, Arnaud C, Zanchetta J, et al. (2001) Effect of parathyroid hormone (1–34) on fractures and bone mineral density in postmenopausal women with osteoporosis. N Engl J Med 344:1434–1441

A99. O'Gradaigh D, Debiram I, Love S, et al. (2003) A prospective study of discordance in diagnosis of osteoporosis using spine and proximal femur bone densitometry. Osteoporos Int 14:13–18

A100. Orwoll E, Ettinger M, Weiss S, et al. (2000) Alendronate for the treatment of osteoporosis in men. N Engl J Med 343:604–610

A101. Orwoll E (2003) Men, bone and estrogen: unresolved issues. Osteoporos Int 14:93–98

A102. Perese E, Perese K (2003) Health problems of women with severe mental illness. J Am Acad Nurse Pract 15:212–219

A103. Peter C, Cook W, Nunamaker D, et al. (1996) Effect of alendronate on fracture healing and bone remodeling in dogs. J Orthop Res 14:74–79

A104. Pfeifer M, Lehmann R, Minne H (2001) Die Therapie der Osteoporose aus dem Blickwinkel einer auf Evidenz basierenden Medizin. Med Klin 96:270–280

A105. Pols H, Felsenberg D, Hanley D, et al. (1999) Multinational, placebo-controlled, randomized trial of the effects of alendronate on bone density and fracture risk in postmenopausal women with low bone mass: results of the FOSIT study. Osteoporos Int 9:461–468

A106. Ralston S (2003) Genetic determinants of susceptibility to osteoporosis. Curr Opin Pharmacol 3:286–290

A107. Rauch F, Plotkin H, Zeitlin L, Glorieux F (2003) Bone mass, size and density in children and adolescence with osteogenesis imperfecta: effect of intravenous pamidronate therapy. J Bone Miner Res 18:610–614

A108. Ravn P, Neugebauer G, Christiansen C (2002) Association between pharmacokinetics of oral ibandronate and clinical response in bone mass and bone turnover in women with postmenopausal osteoporosis. Bone 30:320–324

A109. Recker R, Hinders S, Davies K, et al. (1996) Correcting calcium nutritional deficiency prevents spine fractures in elderly women. J Bone Miner. Res 11:1961–1966

A110. Reginster J, Meuermanns L, Zegels B, et al. (1998) The effect of sodium monofluorophosphate plus calcium on vertebral fracture rate in postmenopausal women with moderate osteoporosis: a randomised controlled trial. Ann Intern Med 129:1–8

A111. Reginster J, Minne H, Sorensen O, et al. (2000) Randomized trial of the effects of risedronate on vertebral fractures in women with established postmenopausal osteoporosis. Osteoporos Int 11:83–91

A112. Reginster J, Meunier P (2003) Strontium ranelate phase 2 dose-ranging studies: PREVOS and STRATOS studies. Osteoporos Int 14(Suppl3):S56–S65

A113. Reid I, Ames R, Evans M, Gamble G, Sharpe S (1995) Long-term effect of calcium supplementation on bone loss and fracture in postmenopausal women: a randomized controlled trial. Am J Med 98:331–335

A114. Reid I, Brown J, Burckhardt P, et al. (2002) Intravenous zoledronic acid in postmenopausal women with low bone mineral density. N Engl J Med 346:653–661

A115. Richy F, Bousquet J, Eherlich G, et al. (2003) Inhaled corticosteroid effects on bone in asthmatic and COPD patients: a quantitative systematic study. Osteoporos Int 14:179–190

A116. Ringe J, Faber H, Dorst A (2001) Alendronate treatment of established primary osteoporosis in men: results of a 3-year prospective study. J Clin Endocrinol Metab 86:5252–5255

A117. Ringe J, Dorst A, Faber H, et al. (2003) Three-monthly ibandronate bolus injection offers favourable tolerability and sustained efficacy advantage over two years in established corticosteroid-induced osteoporosis. Rheumatology 42: 743–749

A118. Rodan G, Martin T (2000) Therapeutic approaches to bone diseases. Science 289:1508–1514

A119. Roschger P, Rinnerthaler S, Yates J, et al. (2001) Alendronate increases degree and uniformity of mineralisation in cancellous bone and decreases the porosity in cortical bone of osteoporotic women. Bone 29:185–191

A120. Rosen C, Bilezikian J (2001) Anabolic therapy of osteoporosis. J Clin Endocrinol Metab 86:957–964

A121. Rubin M., Cosman F, Lindsay R, Bilezikian J (2002) The anabolic effect of parathyroid hormone. Osteoporos Int 13:267–277

A122. Saag K, Emkey R, Schnitzer T, et al. Alendronate for the treatment of glucocorticoid-induced osteoporosis. N Engl J Med 339:292–299

A123. Sambrook P, Kotowicz M, Nash P, et al. (2003) Prevention and treatment of glucocorticoid-induced osteoporosis: a comparison of calcitriol, vitamin D plus calcium and alendronate plus calcium. J Bone Miner Res 18:919–924

A124. Schürch MA, Rizzoli R, Mermillod B, et al. (1996) A prospective study on socioeconomic aspects of fracture of the proximal femur. J Bone Miner Res 11:1935–1942

A125. Seaman E (2003) Reduced bone formation and increased bone resorption: rational targets for the treatment of osteoporosis. Osteoporos Int 14 (Suppl3): S2–S8

A126. Siebler T, Shalet S, Robson H. (2002) Effects of chemotherapy on bone metabolism and skeletal growth. Horm Res 58(Suppl1):80–85

A127. Siminoski K, Fitzgerals A, Flesch G, et al. (2000) Intravenous pamidronate for treatment of reflex sympathetic dystrophy during breast feeding. J Bone Miner Res 15:2052–2055

A128. Sirola J, Kröger H, Honkanen R, et al. (2003) Smoking may impair the bone protective effects of nutritional calcium: a population-based approach. J Bone Miner Res 18:1036–1042

A129. Smith I, Dowsett M (2003) Aromatase inhibitors in breast cancer. N Engl J Med 348:2431–2442

A130. Smith S, Heer M (2002) Calcium and bone metabolism during space flight. Nutrition 18:849–852

A131. Szulc P, Delmas P (2001) Biochemical markers of bone turnover in men. Calcif Tissue Int 69:229–230

A132. Takeda S, Elefteriou F, Levasseur R, et al (2002) Leptin regulates bone formation via the sympathetic nervous system. Cell 111:305–317

A133. Thiébaud D, Burckhardt P, Kriegbaum H, et al. (1997) Three monthly intravenous injections of ibandronate in the treatment of postmenopausal osteoporosis. Am J Med 103:298–307

A134. Tonino R, Meunier P, Emkey R, et al. (2000) Skeletal benefits of alendronate: 7-year treatment of postmenopausal osteoporotic women. J Clin Endocrinol Metab 85:3109–3115

A135. Torgenson D, Bell-Seyer S (2001) Hormone replacement therapy and prevention of nonvertebral fractures: a meta-analysis of randomized trials. JAMA 285:2891–2897

A136. Torgerson D, Dolan P (1998) Prescribing by general practitioners after an osteoporotic fracture. Ann Rheum Dis 57:378–379

A137. Truumees E (2002) The roles of vertebroplasty and kyphoplasty as parts of a treatment strategy for osteoporotic vertebral compression fractures. Curr Opin Orthop 13:193–199

A138. Turner C (2002) Biomechanics of bone: determinants of skeletal fragility and bone quality. Osteoporos Int 13:97–104

A139. Turner C (2002) Mechanotransduction in skeletal cells. Curr Opin Orthop 13:363–367

A140. Van Schoor N, Devillé W, Bouter L, et al. (2002) Acceptance and compliance with external hip protectors: a systematic review of the literature. Osteoporos Int 13:917–924

A141. Van Staa T, Leufkens H, Cooper C (2002) Does a fracture at one site predict later fractures at other sites? A British cohort study. Osteoporos Int 13:624–629

A142. Van Staa T, Leufkens H, Cooper C (2002) The epidemiology of corticosteroid-induced osteoporosis: a meta-analysis. Osteoporos Int 13:777–787

A143. Verrotti A, Greco R Latini G, et al. (2002) Increased bone turnover in prepubertal, pubertal and postpubertal patients receiving carbamazepine. Epilepsia 43:1488–1492

A144. Wallach S, Cohen S, Reid D, et al. (2000) Effects of risedronate treatment on bone density and vertebral fracture in patients on corticosteroid therapy. Calcif Tissue Int 67:277–285

A145. Watts N, Harris S, Genant H, et al. (1990) Intermittent cyclical etidronate treatment of postmenopausal osteoporosis. N Engl J Med 323:73–79

A146. Weber T, Drezner M (2001) Effect of alendronate on bone mineral density in male idiopathic osteoporosis. Metabolism 50:912–915

A147. Women's Health Initiative Group (2002) Risks and benefits of estrogen plus progestin in healthy postmenopausal women. JAMA 288:321–333

A148. Young M (2003) Bone matrix proteins: their function, regulation, and relationship to osteoporosis. Osteoporos Int 14(Suppl3):S35–S42

A149. Zaidi M, Blair H, Moonga B, et al. (2003) Osteoclastogenesis, bone resorption, and osteoclast-based therapeutics. J Bone Miner Res 18:599–609

A150. Zuckerman J, Skovron M, Koval K, et al. (1995) Postoperative complications and mortality associated with operative delay in older patients who have a fracture of the hip. J Bone Joint Surg 77:1551–1556

Selected Articles Recently Published

1. Ahlborg H, Johnell O, Turner C et al. (2003) Bone loss and bone size after menopause. N Engl J Med 349:327-334
2. Black D, Greenspan S, Ensrud K et al. (2003) The effects of parathyroid hormone and alendronate alone or in combination in postmenopausal osteoporosis. N Engl J Med 349:1207-1215
3. Bonewald L (2003) Osteocyte biology. Curr Opin Orthop 14:311-316
4. Cohen A, Shane E (2003) Osteoporosis after solid organ and bone marrow transplantation. Osteoporos Int 14:617-630
5. Damilakis J, Papadokostakis G, Perisinakis K et al. (2003) Can radial bone mineral density and quantitative ultrasound measurements reduce the number of women who need axial density skeletal assessment? Osteoporos Int 14:688-693
6. Finkelstein J, Hayes A, Hunzelman J et al. (2003) The effects of parathyroid hormone, alendronate, or both in men with osteoporosis. N Engl J Med 349:1216-1226
7. Fitzpatrick L, Heaney R (2003) Got soda? J Bone Miner Res 18:1570-1571
8. Frank G (2003) Role of estrogen and androgen in pubertal skeletal physiology. Med Pediatr Oncol 41:217-221
9. Gandrud L, Cheung J, Daniels M, Bachrach L (2003) Low-dose intravenous pamidronate reduces fractures in childhood osteoporosis. Pediatr Endocrinol Metab 16:887-892
10. Gourlay M, Richy F, Reginster J (2003) Strategies for the prevention of hip fractures. Am J Med 115:309-317
11. Hillner B, Chlebowski R, Gralow J et al. (2003) American Society of Clinical Oncology 2003 update on the role of bisphosphonates and bone health issues in women with breast cancer. Clin Oncol Sept 8
12. Jachna C, Whittle J, Lukert B et al. (2003) Effect of hospitalist consultation on treatment of osteoporosis in hip fracture patients. Osteoporos Int 14:665-671
13. Kaufman J, Bolander M, Bunta A et al. (2003) Barriers and solutions to osteoporosis care in patients with a hip fracture. J Bone Joint Surg 85A:1837-1843
14. Khosla S (2003) Parathyroid hormone plus alendronate – a combination that does not add up. N Engl J Med 349:1277-1279
15. McGartland C, Robson P, Murray L et al. (2003) Carbonated soft drink consumption and bone mineral density in adolescence: the Northern Ireland Young Hearts Project. J Bone Miner Res 18:1563-1569
16. Mukherjee A, Shalet S (2003) Growth hormone replacement therapy (GHRT) in children and adolescents: skeletal impact. Med Pediatr Oncol 41:235-242
17. Nordin C (2003) Should the treatment of osteoporosis be more selective? Osteoporos Int 14:99-102
18. Onley R (2003) Regulation of bone mass by growth hormone. Med Pediatr Oncol 41:228-234
19. Orwell E (2003) Men, bone and estrogen: unresolved issues. Osteoporos Int 14:93-98
20. Rehman O, Lane N (2003) Effect of glucocorticoids on bone density. Med Pediatr Oncol 41:212-216

21. Santini D, Vespasiani G, Vincenti B (2003) The antineoplastic role of bisphos-phonates: from basic research to clinical evidence. Ann Oncol 14:1468-1476
22. Seeman E (2003) Periosteal bone formation – a neglected determinant of bone strength. N Engl J Med 349:320-323
23. Stakkestad J, Benevolenskaya L, Stepan J et al. (2003) Intravenous ibandronate injections given every three months: a new treatment option to prevent bone loss in postmenopausal women. Ann Rheum Dis 62:969-975
24. Taguchi A, Sanada M, Krall E et al. (2003) Relationship between dental pan-oramic radiographic findings and biochemical markers of bone turnover. J Bone Miner Res 18:1689-1694
25. Zaidi M, Moonga B, Sun l et al. (2003) Understanding osteoclast formation and function: implications for future therapies for osteoporosis. Curr Opin Orthop 14:341-350

Subject Index

A

A class recommendation   101
abnormalities of bone   28
acetylsalicylic acid   105
acids   92
acitivity   85
acupuncture   106
acute phase   105–106
– reaction   136
adipocytes   11
adolescence   88
aerobics   88
age   42
AIDS-osteopathy   195
alcohol   46
– alcoholism   48
– high alcohol intake   90
aledronate   134, 137–138
alfacalcidol   115
algodystrophy   33
algorithm for diagnostic investigation
    and treatment of osteoporosis   69
alkaline phosphatase (ALP),
    bone-specific   76, 196
allendronate   137
ALP (alkaline phosphatase),
    bone-specific   76, 196
aluminium   48, 196
– deposition   196
aluminium-containing antacids   212
alveolar bone   52
Alzheimer's disease   197
aminobisphosphonates   128, 188
AML (acute myeloid leukaemia)   194
amyloidosis   195

amytrophic lateral sclerosis   197
anabolic steroids   127
anaesthetics, local   106
analgetics   105
anastrozole   208
androgens   12, 17–18
andropause   174
ankle   67
anorexia nervosa   45
antacids, aluminium-containing   212
antiacids   48
antiandrogens   209
anticoagulants   48, 94
anticonvulsants   94, 212
antiresorptives   148
antiretroviral therapy (HAART)   195
aortic insufficiency   188
apoptosis   5, 149
aromatase inhibitors   207
aromates   17
arthritis
– osteoarthritis   53, 89
– primary chronic polyarthritis (PCP)
    95, 198
arthrosis, spondylarthroses   54
aseptic loosening of prosthesis
    169–173
asthma bronchiale   198, 200
atrophy   14
– of bone   38
autoimmune disorders   200

B

Baastrup syndrome   52
back pain   49, 54
– acute   51–52
ballooning   53
barbiturates   94
basic muticellular unit (BMU)   10
beclomethasone dipropionate   202
biconcavity   53
biliary cirrhosis, primary   192
biochemical markers of bone turnover
  76
biomechanical properties   28
– extrinsic   28
– intrinsic   28
biopsy
– bone   22, 54, 142, 149, 197, 212, 217
– iliac crest   38, 79
– needles   39
bisphosphonates   128–144, 184,
  216–218
– contraindications   135, 137
– intravenous application   218
– monitoring effects of   142–143
– nonresponders to   143–144
– oral bisphosphonates   137
– pharmacokinetics   134–135
– toxicity   135–137
bleeding, vaginal   123
blockade of the stellar plexus   216
blood
– pressure   92
– vessels   11
blue sclerae   51, 188
BMC (bone mineral content)   60
BMD (bone mineral density)   8, 58–72
– indications   68–70
– radiation dose   71–72
– techniques for measuring BMD   59
BMP (bone morphogenic proteins)   6
body weight
– ideal   93
– low   45
– underweight   93
bone   5–23
– abnormalities   28
– adynamic   196–197

– alkaline phosphatase (ALP),
  bone-specific   76, 196
– alveolar   52
– atrophy   38
– balance   14
– cancellous bone   8
– biopsy   22, 54, 142, 149, 197, 212, 217
– cells   11
– compact bone   8
– cortical bone   8
– electric potentials in bone   107–108
– formation, parameters of   76
– frozen   128
– interdependence of bone
  and marrow (scheme)   11
– malignant bone lesions   54
– markers of bone turnover   75–79
– marrow   206
– mass   8
– – peak adult bone mass (PABM)
  25
– – peak bone mass   22
– matrix proteins   5
– microarchitecture   66
– mineral content (see BMC)   60
– mineral density (see BMDs)
  8, 58–72
– morphogenic proteins (BMPs)   6
– phantom bone   217
– quality of bone   27
– remodelling units (BRU)   13
– resorption, parameters of   76
– robbers   90–93
– scan (see also sonography/
  ultrasound)   56, 105, 215
– sialoprotein (BSP)   5, 77
– spongy bone   8
– strength   133
– structural bone unit   16
– trabecular bone (see there)   8–9, 65
– tubular bone   27
– turnover (see there)   28, 38
– vanishing bone disease
  (Gorham-Stout syndrome)   35, 217
robbers, bone   90–93
boron   83
breast cancer   123, 206–209
– hypogonadism with breast cancer
  206–209

breathing exercises, deep breathing
   106
bronchial
– asthma   198, 200
– cancer   198
BRUs (bone remodelling units)   13
BSP (bone sialoprotein)   5, 77
BUA (broad-band ultrasound
   attenuation)   65
budesonide   202

C

caffeine   90
calcaneus   66
calcification   54
calcitonin   106, 151, 184
calcitriol   115, 149, 184
calcium   80–83, 109–112, 188
– chelated   111
– children   184, 188
– deposits   152
– diet, calcium-rich   80
– excretion of   77
– hypercalcemia   111, 128
– hypocalcemia   136
– intake   45, 81
– naturally derived   110
– recommendation for adults   109
– refined calcium carbonate   111
– salts   110
– supplements of   110
– tablets   83
callus formation, hyperplastic   188
canaliculi   12
cancellous bone   8
cancer (see also tumours)
– breast (see there)   123, 206–209
– bronchial   198
– prostate   127, 178–179
carbamazepine   48, 94
cardiology   190–192
– chronic cardiac insufficiency   95
cardiovascular diseases   89
carrying of load   85
castration   176
cement lines   8
cheeses   82

children/childhood   71, 80, 88, 114,
   180–189
– mechanism of osteoporosis
   in children   184
– WHO definition   181
cholestyramine   212
christmas tree phenomenon   52
chronic phase   106–107
– long term   107
– short term   106
cigarette smoking   46
cirrhosis, primary biliary   192
clodronate   140, 208
CML (chronic myeloid leukaemia)
   194
Coca Cola   91
colestipol   212
colitis ulcerosa   192
collagen   5–7
Colles’ fractures   32, 167
compact cortical bone   8
complex regional pain syndrome
   (CRPS)   33, 215
computed tomography (see CT)
   56, 64
contraceptives   47
copper   83
cortical bone   8
corticosteroids   200
– inhalation therapy (ICS)   202
– osteoporosis, corticosteroid-induced
   199–200
cortisone   16
costs, monetary   3
COX-2-inhibitor   106
Crohn’s disease   182, 192, 200, 204
cross-linking   28
– telopeptides, cross-linked   76
CRPS (complex regional pain
   syndrome)   33, 215
CT (computed tomography)   56
– 3 dimensional (volumetric) imaging
   (3D-CT)   65
– quantitative (see QCT)   64
CTX-CROSSLAPS   77
Cushing’s syndrome   182, 192, 199
cyclosporin A   48, 205
cystic fibrosis   198
cytokines   12, 19, 217

D

3D-CT (3 dimensional [volumetric] imaging) 65
Daidzein 125
deafness 188
deep breathing exercises 106
definition of osteoporosis 24–32
deformity grading system 30
degree of severity 37
dehydroepiandrosterone (DHEA) 126
demineralisation, periosteocytic 39
densitrometry, International Society of Clinical Densitometry (ISCD) 62
depression 45
desferal tests 196
desoxypyridinoline 76
DEXA, DXA (dual energy X-ray absorptiometry) 60–61
DHEA (dehydroepiandrosterone) 126
diabetes mellitus 95, 192, 195
– neuropathy, diabetic 197
– steroid-induced 204
disc degeneration 53
diseases (see syndromes / diseases)
Dowager's hump 52
doxorubicin 210
drugs/medications 93–94, 104–105, 199–213
– immunouppressive 48
– list of 199
– osteoporomalacia, drug-induced 211–213
DXA, DEXA (dual energy X-ray absorptiometry) 60–61
– DXA unit 60
– full body DXA scanner 61

E

edematous processes 57
electric potentials in bone 107–108
emboli, pulmonary 123
empty box 53
endocrinology 192

endoprosthesis 169–173
– aseptic loosening of prosthesis 169–173
– micromovements 170
– polyethylene 170
– tissue compatibility of the implant 170
endosteal
– envelope 8
– lining cells 13
endosteum 26
endothelial cells 11
energy balance 21
epilepsy 197
ER (oestrogen receptors) 12, 124, 146
etidronate 137, 139, 212
European Prospective Osteoporosis Study (EPOS) 175
evidence-based medicine 97
excessive sport 44
exemestane 208
exercise 87–88
– weight-bearing 88
exostoses 152
extreme sports 89

F

falling
– main causes of falls in the elderly 156
– risc factors for falls 155
– tendency to fall 48
fast losers 200
fat cells 17
fatique
– damage 10
– fracture 29
fatty acids 47
femoral neck 31
– length 31
– width 31
femur, proximal 56
fibronectin 5
fingers 64
FIT (fracture intervention trial) study 137

FK506 (tacrolimus)   205
fluoride   83, 151–152, 196, 213
fluorosis   54, 152
folic acid   85
foreign body granulomas   171
fracture   2–3, 29, 155–173
– Colles' fractures   32, 167
– fatique   29
– FIT (fracture intervention trial)
   study   137
– fracture sites   161
– fragility   29
– of the hip   2, 31–32, 161
– of the humerus   168
– low trauma   29
– management of osteoporotic
   fractures   160
– microfracture   10, 27, 105
– osteoporotic   3
– pathologic   29
– previous   43
– repair   136
– risk factors for osteoporotic fracture
   158
– vertebral (spinal)   29–31, 55, 164
– wrist   32, 167–168
fragility   28
– fracture   29
frozen bone   128
fruit juice   81–82
fruits   82

G

gap junctions   12
gardening   88
gastric operations   193
gastroenterology/gastrointestinal
   complaints   135, 192–193
Gaucher's disease   193–194
genetics   40, 193
genistein   125
GH (growth hormones)   16, 184
glucocorticoids/glucocorticoid therapy
   47, 94, 196, 198, 200–201, 212
glycoproteins   5
GnRH (gonadotropin-releasing-hor-
   monc)   207

gold standard   60
gonarthrosis   52
Gorham-Stout syndrome
   (vanishing bone disease)   35, 217
grading of osteoporosis, clinical   37
growth
– factors   153
– hormones (GH)   16
guidelinse for safe movement   87

H

HAART (antiretroviral therapy)   195
hair   52–53
– increased hair growth   215
height, loss of   52, 55
hemangiomatosis   217
hematology   193–194
hematopoietic cells   11
hemiplegia   44
hemochromatosis   176
hemolytic conditions, congenital   194
heparin   194
heparin   48, 94, 194
hepatic disorders, chronic   123
HERS study   122
hip
– fracture   2, 31–32, 161
– joint   67
histamines   194
histological parameters   38
histomorphometry/histomorpho-
   metric parameters   79, 197
HIV infection   195
Hodgkin's disease   209
hormones   12, 16
– gonadotropin-releasing-hormone
   (GnRH)   207
– growth (GH)   16, 184
– hormone replacement therapy
   (HRT)   117–127
– parathyroid (PTH)   12, 16
– thyroid (TH)   12, 16
hot flashes   145
housework   85
HPT (hyperparathyroidism)   54, 196
HRT (hormone replacement therapy)
   117–127

humerus fractures   168
hydroxyapatite mass   64
hydroxyproline   77
hypercalcemia (see also calcium)   111,
    128
hypercalciuria   188
hyperparathyroidism (HPT)   54
– primary (pHPT)   192
– secondary (sHPT)   196
hyperplastic callus formation   188
hypertension   22, 123
hyperthyroidism   192
hypertrigyceridemia   123
hypocalcemia   136
hypogonadism   126, 176, 192, 209
– secondary   206
hypophosphatemia   212
hypothalamus   21

I

ibandronate   135, 139–140
ICS (inhalation corticosteroid therapy)
    200
ifosfamid   210
IGF binding proteins   201
IJO (idiopathic juvenile osteoporosis)
    35, 185
iliac creast biopsy   38, 79
immobilisation   19, 44, 184, 198, 206
– inactivity (immobilisation osteo-
    porosis)   33
immunohistology/immunohistological
    techniques   39, 79
immunosuppression   205
– drugs, immunosuppressive   48, 196
implant, tissue compatibility of   170
inactivity (immobilisation osteo-
    porosis)   33
– chronic   43
infectious disorders   195
inflammatory bowel disease   95
infractions   29
insulin   16
interdisciplinary approach   189
International Society of Clinical
    Densitometry (ISCD)   62

intestinal operations   193
intracortical envelope   8
intraosseous pressure   105
intravenous therapy   140
involutional (age-related, type II)
    osteoporosis   36
ischemic attacks, transient   197
isoflavones   124
isoniazide   48

J

joint pain   198
juvenile idiopathic osteoporosis   35

K

Kallmann syndrome   176
keratoconus   188
kidney
– stones   115, 188
– transplantation   195
kissing spine   52
Klinefelter's syndrome   126, 176
knots   28
kyphoplasty   167
kyphosis   52

L

laboratory investigations   73–79
– screening tests   73
lactation   43, 81
lactose intolerance   192
lacunae   12
least significant change (LSC)   78
legumes   124
LEPS (lower extremity pain syndrome)
    152
leptin   12, 20–22, 152
letrozole   208
leukaemia
– acute myeloid (AML)   194
– chronic myeloid (CML)   194
lifting of load   85

lignans   124
lining cells   11
lipid   47, 92
lithium   48
load
– carrying   85
– lifting   85
– mechanical loading   20
local anaesthetics   106
Looser's zones   29, 39, 54, 196
LSC (least significant change)   78
lumbar vertebrae   67
lying down   85
lymphangiomatosis   217
lymphoma   57
– malignant   194, 200, 209

M

magnesium   83, 116
– hypomagnesemia   136
magnetic
– field therapy   107
– resonance imaging (MRI)   33, 57,
   214
malabsorption syndromes   192
Male Turner (Noonan) syndrome   176
malignant
– bone lesions   54
– lymphoma   194, 200, 209
– melanoma   123
manganese   83
marathon runners   29
markers of bone turnover   75–79
– biochemical markers   76
mast cells   11, 194
mastocytosis, systemic   194
matrix   5
mechanical loading   20
mechanoreceptor   20
mechanosensory cells   13
medical history   50
medications (see also drugs)   93–94,
   104–105
men, osteoporosis in   174–179
– prevention of   178
menopause

– male   177
– postmenopausal (type I) osteoporosis   35
metacarpals   56
metalloproteins   6
metamizol   105
metastases   57, 75, 198
– osseous   128
methotrexate   210
mevalonic acid metabolism   132
microarchitecture   28
microdamage   10
microfracture   10, 27, 105
microgravity   44
micromovements   170
microradioscopy   56
migration   171
milk / milk products   81–82
mineral
– content (see BMC bone mineral
   content)   60
– density (see BMDs bone mineral
   density)   8, 58–72
– water   82
mineralisation   6–7
– primary   6
– secondary   7
minerals   5, 47
mitral valve, prolapse of   188
modelling   9
monetary costs   3
monitoring   78
– effects of bisphosphonates   142–143
MORE (multiple outcomes of raloxifene evaluation) study   145
MRI (magnetic resonance imaging)
   33, 57, 214
multiple
– outcomes of raloxifene evaluation
   (MORE) study   145
– sclerosis   197
muscle
– relaxants   106
– tone   51
MXA (morphometric X-ray absorptiometry)   55
myeloma   57
– multiple   193, 200

N

nandrolone   127
National Osteoporosis Foundation
    (NOF)   67, 69, 87, 93–94, 96, 117, 199
needles for biopsy   39
nephrolithiasis   111
nephrology   195–197
neridronate   140
neurology   197
neurons   21
neuropathy, diabetic   197
NOF (National Osteoporosis Foun-
    dation)   67, 69, 87, 93–94, 96, 117, 199
nonresponders to bisphosphonates
    143–144
nonsteroidal antirheumatic drugs
    105
Noonan (Male Turner) syndrome
    176
noradrenalin   21
NTX-OSTEOMARK   76
nutritional deficiency   47

O

obesity   93
obstacles   48
OC (osteocalcin)   5, 76, 84, 116
ocular reactions   136
oesophagitis   135
oestrogen   12, 16, 18, 23, 118, 120,
    123–126
– analogues   120
– natural   123–126
– – found in soy   125
– phyto-oestrogens   123
– receptors (ER)   12, 124, 146
– – oestrogen receptor modulator
    (see SERM)   145–147
OFELY-study   155
OI (osteogenesis imperfecta)   185,
    187–189
– Osteogenesis Imperfecta Founda-
    tion (OIF)   189
– types   188
ointments   94

oncology   198
operations, gastric and intestinal   193
OPG (osteoprotegerin)   19, 196
opiate   106
orchidectomy   209
orchitis, status post-orchitis   176
organ transplants   200
osseous metastases   128
osteitis fibrosa cystica   196
osteoanabolic therapy   148
osteoarthritis   54, 89
osteoblasts   11–12
osteocalcin (OC)   5, 76, 84, 116
osteoclast   11
– activity   16
osteocytes   11–12
osteodystrophy, renal (ROD)   79, 195
osteogenesis imperfecta (see OI)   185,
    187–189
osteoid   11, 84
osteology   4
osteolytic lesions / syndromes   35, 198
osteomalacia   29, 38, 49, 54, 134, 193,
    196
osteonecrosis   214
osteonectin   5, 76
osteopenia   26
osteopontin   5
osteoporomalacia   94, 193
– drug-induced   211–213
osteoporosis
– algorithm for diagnostic investiga-
    tion and treatment of osteoporosis
    69
– clinical grading   37
– corticosteroid-induced   199
– definition   24–32
– European Prospective Osteoporosis
    Study (EPOS)   175
– fracture, osteoporotic (see there)
    2–3, 29, 155–173
– inactivity (immobilisation osteo-
    porosis)   33
– idiopathic osteoporosis
– – juvenile (IJO)   35, 185
– – young adults   35
– involutional (age-related, type II)
    osteoporosis   36

– in men   174–179
– National Osteoporosis Foundation
  (NOF)   67, 69, 87, 93–94, 96, 117,
  199
– osteoporosis tummy   52
– pain, osteoporotic (see there)
  105–108
– postmenopausal (type I) osteoporosis   35
– preventive care   80–96
– primary   190
– secondary   190
– transient (transitory)   33, 57, 214
– transplantation (see there)
  204–205
– treatment   97–104
– tumour therapy-induced   206–213
osteoprotegerin (OPG)   19, 196
osteosclerotic lesions   198
over-acidification   93

P

PABM (peak adult bone mass)   25
Paget's disease   75, 128, 172
pain
– back pain (see there)   49, 51–52, 54
– complex regional pain syndrome
  (CRPS)   33, 215
– joint pains   198
– lower extremity pain syndrome
  (LEPS)   152
– management of pain   105–108
– osteoporotic   105
– sympathetically maintained pain
  (SMP)   215
pamidronate   140
pancreatic insufficiency   192
paracetamol   105
paralysis   44
paraplegia   44
parathyroid hormones/parathormone
  (PTH)   12, 16, 148–150, 196
parathormone-related proteins
  (PTHrP)   198
parathyroidectomy   197
Parkinson's disease   48, 197

PCP (primary chronic polyarthritis)
  95, 198
peak bone mass   22
– peak adult bone mass (PABM)   25
perforations   27
periosteal envelope   8
periosteocytic demineralisation   39
phalanges by ultrasound   198
phantom bone   217
phenytoin   94, 212
pheobarbital   212
phosphate   92
phosphorus   83
pHPT (primary hyperparathyroidism)
  192
physical examination   50
physiotherapy   107
phyto-oestrogens   123
PICP and PINC (propeptides of type I
  procollagen)   76
picture frame   53
piezolectricity   107
pigmentation of the skin   215
pitfalls   63
plexus, blockade of the stellar plexus
  216
polyarthritis, primary chronic (PCP)
  95, 198
polycythemia vera (PV)   194
polyethylene   170
polymethylmethacrylate (PMMA)
  167
postmenopausal (type I) osteoporosis
  35
posture   51
Prader-Willi syndrome   176
prednisone   94, 200
pregnancy   43, 81
preventive care   80–96
– prevention of osteoporosis in men
  178
primary osteoporosis   190
progestin   120
prolactinomas   176
propeptides of type I procollagen
  (PICP and PINC)   76
proper sitting   86
propranolol   22

prostaglandins   19, 105, 153
- prostaglandin E   200, 216
prostate
- cancer/carcinoma   127, 178–179
- hypertrophy, prostatic   127
- malignancy, prostatic   209
prostate-specific antigen (PSA)   127
prosthesis (see endoprosthesis)
  169–173
proteins   47, 92
PSA (prostate-specific antigen)   127
PTH (parathyroid hormones/
  parathormone)   12, 16, 148–150, 196
- osteoanabolic action   148
- PTH2 receptor   149
PTHrP (parathormone-related proteins)   198
pulmonology / pulmonary   198
- chronic pulmonary diseases   95
- emboli   123
PV (polycythemia vera)   194
pyrophosphate   129

Q

QCT (quantitative computer
  tomography)   64
- wrist (pQCT)   64
quality of bone   27
QUI (quantitative ultrasound index)
  66
QUS (quantitative ultrasound
  sonography)   65

R

RA (radiographic absorptiometry)
  65
race   41–42
radiation dose, MMD   71–72
radiographic absorptiometry (RA)
  65
radiolucent lines   171
radiotherapy   206
radius   67
raloxifene   145–147
- multiple outcomes of raloxifene
  evaluation (MORE) study   145
- use for the heart (RUTH) trial   146
RANK/RANKL signalling pathway   12
RDA (recommended daily allowance)
  47
recommendations
- A class recommendation   101
- calcium, recommendations for
  adults   109
- RDA (recommended daily
  allowance)   47
reflex dystrophy, sympathetic   33
region of interest (ROI)   64
rehabilitation   160
remodelling   9–10, 15, 26
- bone remodelling units (BRU)   13
- cycle   13, 15
renal
- insufficiency   95, 111
- osteodystrophy (ROD)   79, 195
repair phase   166
rheumatology/rheumatic disorders
  198, 200
Ricket's disease   114
rifampicin   212
risc factors   176
- for falls   155
rise and walk test   48
risedronate   134, 137–139
risk factors   40–48
- for osteoporotic fracture   158
ROD (renal osteodystrophy)   79, 195
ROI (region of interest)   64
ruffled border   11
rugger-jersey-spine   54, 196
RUTH (raloxifene use for the heart)
  trial   146

S

salt   92
- calcium salts   110
sarcopenia   174
Schmorl's nodes   30, 53
sclerae
- blue   51, 188

– rupture 188
scleroses, subchondral 54
SD (standard deviation) 63
secondary osteoporosis 190
self-help measures 80
SERM (oestrogen receptor modulator)
 145–147
– SERM's action 146
severity, degree of 37
sex 42
sialoprotein, bone (BSP) 5, 77
singh index 31, 55
single energy X-ray absorptiometry
 (SXA) 64
sitting, propper 86
skeletal X-ray 53
skeleton 5, 9
– appendicular 9
– axial 9
– whole 68
skin 52–53
– allergy 136
– pigmentation of 215
sleeping 85
smoking 46, 89–90
– cigarette 46
SMP (sympathetically maintained
 pain) 215
solid tumour 198
sonography / ultrasound
– attenuation of sound 65
– – broad-band ultrasound attenuation (BUA) 65
– bone scan 56, 105, 215
– phalanges by ultrasound 198
– quantitative ultrasound index (QUI)
 66
– quantitative ultrasound sonography
 (QUS) 65
– speed of sound (SOS) 65
sound (see also sonography/
 ultrasound)
– attenuation of sound 65
– – broad-band ultrasound attenuation (BUA) 65
– speed of sound (SOS) 65
spine
– deformity index 55

– kissing spine 52
– rugger-jersey-spine 54
– vertebral (spinal) fractures 29–31,
 55, 164
– – midthoracic area 164
spondylarthroses 54
spondylitis 54
spongy bone 8
sports, excessive/extreme 44, 89
sprays 94
standard deviation (SD) 63
statin 153
status post-orchitis 176
stellar plexus, blockade of 216
steroid-induced diabetes mellitus
 204
stress lines 107
stroke 197
strontium 83, 153–154
structural bone unit 16
subchondral scleroses 54
Sudeck's disease 33, 57, 214
sugar 91
sunlight exposure 212 113
swelling and warmth 215
swimmers/swimming 88
SXA (single energy X-ray absorptiometry) 64
sympathetic / sympathetically
– maintained pain (SMP) 215
– reflex dystrophy 33
symptoms 49
syndromes/diseases
– Alzheimer 197
– Baastrup 52
– Crohn 182, 192, 200, 204
– Cushing 182, 192, 199
– Gaucher 193–194
– Gorham-Stout 35, 217
– Hodgkin 209
– Kallmann 176
– Klinefelter 126, 176
– Male Turner (Noonan) 176
– Paget 75, 128, 172
– Parkinson 48, 197
– Prader-Willi 176
– Ricket 114
– Sudeck 33, 57, 214

T

tacrolimus (FK506)   205
tamoxifen   207–208
teenagers   80
teeth   52–53
– anomalies   188
telopeptides, cross-link   76
tendency to fall   48
tennis players   88
testosterone   18, 126–127
– deficiency   176
– enanthate   178
– replacement therapy   126, 174
tetracyclins   154
TH (thyroid hormones)   12, 16, 48, 94
thermography   215
thoracolumbar junction   164
thrombospondin-2   6
thrombotic tendency   123
thyroid hormones (TH)   12, 16, 48, 94
tibolone   120
tissue compatibility of the implant
   170
trabecular bone   8–9
– architecture   65
trace elements   116
trajection lines   107
transcriptional
– genes   20
– regulation   20
transient
– ischemic attacks   197
– (transitory) osteoporosis   33, 57, 214
transplantation
– organs   200
– – kidney   195
– osteoporosis   204–205
trauma fracture, low   29
treatment of osteoporosis   97–104
– drugs/medications   93–94, 104–105
– treatment strategy   103, 211
triamcinolone   202
trochanter   31
T-score   64
tubular bone   27
tummy, osteoporosis tummy   52
tumours (see also cancer)

– malignancies, prostatic   209
– metastases (see there)   57, 75, 128,
   198
– osteoporosis, tumour therapy-
   induced   206–213
– solid   198
turnover
– high   14, 75
– low   14, 38, 75
two-phase-component   6

U

ultrasound (see sonography/
   ultrasound)   56, 65
underweight   93
unusual local manifestations   214–218
upright posture   86

V

vaginal bleeding   123
vanishing bone disease (Gorham-Stout
   syndrome)   35, 217
vascular disease   19
VDS (vertebral deformation score)   55
vegetables   82
vertebral (spinal)
– column   51
– deformities   30
– – VDS (vertebral deformation
   score)   55
– fractures   29–31, 55
– lumbar vertebrae   67
vertebroplasty   167
verticalisation   53
vibration   20
vision, reduced   48
vitamins   20, 47, 84–85, 112–116
– vitamin A   85, 116
– vitamin B12   85
– vitamin C   84
– vitamin D   84, 112–115, 196
– – children   184, 188
– – metabolism   113, 115
– vitamin K   84, 116

W

walk test   48
walking   88
Ward's triangle   31
warfarin   48, 94
weight-bearing exercises   88
weightlifters   88
wheat products   82
WHO (World health organisation)
    24–26, 181
– osteoporosis in children,
    WHO definition   181
Wolff's law   87
women's health initiative study   118,
    122
wrist
– fractures   32, 167–168
– pQCT   64

X

X-ray   105, 215
– dual energy X-ray absorptiometry
    (DEXA, DXA)   60–61
– morphometric X-ray absorptiome-
    try (MXA)   55
– single energy X-ray absorptiometry
    (SXA)   64
– skeletal   53

Y

yoga   106

Z

zinc   83
zoledronate   135, 140
Z-score   64